I04814O1

Edward Long
850 Lincoln Dr #152
Idaho Falls, Idaho
83401

11 Oct 88

Doctor, WHY *Am I So* TIRED?

Doctor, WHY *Am I So* TIRED?

Richard N. Podell, M.D., F.A.C.P.

PHAROS BOOKS
A SCRIPPS HOWARD COMPANY
NEW YORK

Cover and interior design: Elyse Strongin

Distributed in the United States by Ballantine Books, a division of Random House, Inc., and in Canada by Random House of Canada, Ltd.

Library of Congress Cataloging-in-Publication Data

Podell, Richard N., 1942-
Doctor, why am I so tired?

Bibliography: p.
Includes index.
1. Fatigue—Popular works. I. Title [DNLM:
1. Fatigue—etiology—popular works. WB 146 P742d]
RB150.F37P63 1988 87-60161
Pharos Books ISBN: 0-88687-321-5
Ballantine Books ISBN: 0-345-34878-8

Printed in the United States of America

Pharos Books
A Scripps Howard Company
200 Park Avenue
New York, NY 10166

10 9 8 7 6 5 4 3 2 1

DEDICATION

To my parents with love and appreciation, and with respect and affection to the memory of Solomon A. Berson, M.D., Rishon M. Bialer, HMS '68, and John H. Knowles, M.D.

A WORD FOR THE READER

The information in this book is based on the most recent research, and every attempt has been made to assure that it is totally accurate. However, as new discoveries appear current "facts" may fall into dispute. Therefore, it is important that you check with your doctor before implementing any of the suggestions or recommendations found in this book. Indeed, even assuming the accuracy of each fact, the advice in any book of this nature must anticipate typical or representative situations. Yet each reader and his or her circumstances are unique. Again, your personal physician is the adviser best qualified to help you adapt the general to the specific—to tailor the advice in this book to your personal needs.

ACKNOWLEDGMENTS

My deep appreciation goes to my editors, Beverly Jane Loo, who encouraged this effort, and Hana Lane, who saw it to fruition; Leonard H. Gross, whose criticisms and corrections enormously improved the original manuscript; my literary agent, Pam Bernstein of the William Morris Agency, and my wife, Patricia, for perceptive reading, loving support, and heroic forbearance.

My heartfelt thanks to those who, by reading and responding to portions of the book, helped me improve my understanding of fatigue and communicate it more clearly: Arthur Chotin, Betsy Chotin, Louis Gary, Bernice Heilbrunn Potvin, Sandy Kaldor, Beverly La Puma, Joel Nisenbaum, Florence Podell, Deborah Schrenzel, Steven Schrenzel, Reggie Yoskowitz.

I appreciate the invaluable assistance of the staffs of the Overlook Hospital Medical Library, Cottage Computer, and Word Perfect. Particular thanks go to my skilled, compassionate, and extremely supportive office colleagues: David K. Brown, M.D., Sally Karas, R.N., Jody Geller, R.N., Marjorie Knickerbocker, R.N., Terry McGuirk, Lynn Mason, Robin Ford, Nora Cielo, M.S., Lorrie Katz, R.D.

Of particular importance to me are my teachers who over the years served as mentors and role models: Drs. Leona Baumgartner, Solomon Berson, William Castle, Mort Cohan, Kurt Deuschle, Stanley Gitlow, Donald Kent, Benjamin Josephson, Eleanor Lehman, Joseph Lieberman, James R. Nelson, William Rea, Paul Russell, David Rutstein, Jeanette Simmons, Frank Snope, Anne R. Somers, Colston Warne.

A special thanks to the staff at Pharos Books: David Hendin, publisher and editorial director; H.L. Kirk, who did the copy editing, and Elyse Strongin who supervised the artistic design.

Most important to me are my patients who have shared with me their hopes and fears.

CONTENTS

FOREWORD

In the recent past, there has been a proliferation of excellent lay-oriented books designed to foster public awareness about various aspects of disease. A few have been written by former patients, whereas most have been written by medical professionals. Almost all of these books emphasize the key role that lifestyle choices make in fostering or preventing disease. Unlike other similar works, however, *Doctor, Why Am I So Tired?*, by Dr. Richard N. Podell, focuses on chronic tiredness, a complaint that, even when taken seriously by the medical profession, can be extremely hard to combat. One reason why physicians are often reluctant to deal with the specter of fatigue is that they themselves are bewildered by its overwhelming variety of causes, which run the gamut from well-defined physical factors (glandular deficiency, circulatory or pulmonary disorders, etc.) to subjective factors such as depression and stress.

Although chronic fatigue, per se, is usually regarded as a symptom rather than a treatable condition, it can have as devastating an effect on the patient's quality of life as the most concrete surgical disorder. Since fatigue is hardly life-threatening, however, and since it is a condition that even healthy persons frequently experience, it is tempting to regard tiredness as simply being part of the human condition. Moreover, the problem can be so insidious that it often remains undefined. Because chronic fatigue is a subject that may not be regarded seriously by the medical profession, patients with this complaint are particularly vulnerable to unscientific methods of treatment. This book provides sound, sensitive advice about controversial treatments and theories such as medical hypnosis, orthomolecular nutrition, food allergies, and the Candida yeast theory of fatigue.

Like other works of its kind, *Doctor, Why Am I So Tired?* reflects an encouraging public trend toward the assumption of personal responsibility in preventing serious illness. It urges the patient to take an active role in overcoming his or her condition, without usurping or minimizing the role of the physician. By delineating the many causes of fatigue, the book helps narrow the range of possibilities and eliminate false leads, thus enabling the patient to give a better medical history. More important, by emphasizing the fact that tiredness can be controlled (often merely by means of a simple change in lifestyle), the book reassures affected patients that they need not continue to suffer needlessly.

Doctor, Why Am I So Tired? should be helpful not only to interested lay readers but also to family practitioners, internists, psychologists, and others who treat a wide spectrum of mind/body problems.

Denton A. Cooley, M.D.
Surgeon-in-Chief
Texas Heart Institute

PREFACE

Americans make ten million doctor visits each year seeking relief from feelings of tiredness, weakness, or fatigue, often with little success. Many more people function below par without seeking help, accepting weariness as their way of life. Fatigue is a widespread and life-robbing condition. It impairs work and reduces life's pleasures. I know from professional experience that people plagued with fatigue can be helped.

This book shows how and will arm you with more facts about fatigue than most doctors receive in medical school. It will teach you to select the facts relevant to you and how to communicate them clearly to your doctor. It will help you solve the mystery of why you feel tired, and what you can do about it.

Doctors often do not take the complaint of tiredness seriously. They see it as a "complaint" rather than as a treatable condition. Their attitude is "You're tired? . . . . Who isn't!" They feel fully occupied taking care of concrete illnesses and are impatient with elusive symptoms such as fatigue.

More sympathetic physicians appreciate that weariness can be a sign of many disorders. They may pursue one or two clinical hunches. But when the conditions they're looking for aren't found, patients are often dismissed with "Don't worry. There's nothing really wrong" or "It's all in your head"—adding shame to an already wretched state.

In recent years, I have treated many people who suffer from fatigue. Many asked the same question: "Doctor, why am I tired so much of the time?" Finding the causes of their fatigue and restoring their peak energy has been very gratifying and led me to want to share what I have learned about fatigue and how to combat it.

The first step toward understanding fatigue is recognizing that it has many causes. The one-easy-treatment-for-everybody approach is seductive but does a disservice to most people—whether the magical answer is the traditional "It's all in your head" or the anti-establishment's hypoglycemia, megavitamins, food allergy, and the like.

Step two is appreciating that the main causes of fatigue are few enough (about thirty) for you and your doctor to check for them all *if* you analyze your fatigue problem in an organized way. This book will help organize your knowledge about your fatigue, comparing your personal health history with the symptoms of each condition that can cause chronic tiredness. At the same time, you will learn how to communicate the key points of your history effectively to your physician.

The third and most important step is deciding to take the helm and guide the course of your health care. You will generate a list of the most likely causes of your fatigue. Even though your doctor may need to revise it, your own list of "prime suspects" is an excellent starting point. You are responsible for other decisions as well: which doctor to choose; which diagnostic procedures to accept; weighing the benefits and risks of each proposed treatment.

This active role is *not* medical self-treatment. You should not make health decisions without discussing them with your physician. Incomplete knowledge is dangerous. However, you *must* develop enough confidence to be informed about every aspect of your care. Too much is at stake, and much can be missed or go wrong. Be fair to yourself. Ultimately, you—the fatigue sufferer—must be in charge.

Consider three examples* of people, burdened with unremitting fatigue, who were exhausted still further and brought close to despair by fruitless medical pursuits. They had to persist to find a cure while barely having the stamina to fulfill their jobs and personal responsibilities. Each could have benefited from enlightened self-direction.

Roseann went to her internist because she felt "worn out." He had treated her for a respiratory infection two months earlier. It cleared up, but continuing sinus pain and morning stuffiness made the doctor suspect a lingering infection. Roseann took a full course of antibiotic but was still functioning in low gear a few weeks later. The physician tried a different antibiotic. When that did no good, he suggested she take a vacation. The internist had made a good start, but he gave up.

Soon afterward, Roseann saw her gynecologist for her annual exam. The gynecologist did a blood test and encountered the reason for Roseann's fatigue—iron-deficiency anemia, common among menstruating women. This doctor prescribed the correct treatment: "iron pills." Roseann got her strength back, thanks to an alert physician who didn't dismiss her with "There's nothing wrong."

Martin's doctor pursued the false lead of a physical problem while a serious psychological illness went unrecognized. A fifty-one-year-old businessman, Martin was a sober, recovering alcoholic who felt so tired

* All case histories presented in this book are a composite of various patients with similar medical symptoms. No real names are used.

he could hardly get out of bed in the morning. His doctor's first suspicion was cirrhosis of the liver as a result of Martin's earlier drinking. The physician arranged to have Martin admitted to a hospital for a liver biopsy—taking samples of tissue through a needle passed into the liver.

Martin was worried. He had started a new job and was terrified that co-workers who processed insurance forms would see a diagnosis related to alcoholism. He resolved to pay these medical expenses himself even though his savings were meager.

The past years had been difficult. He had tried desperately to sustain a dying business. Without intending to defraud anyone, he found himself spending the better part of each day dodging creditors. He constantly sought ways to earn extra money, but overdue payables snowballed. After two years he was bailed out by his new employer, who took Martin's good accounts and gave him a job in exchange. A bankruptcy filing shed his liabilities, but not his shame. After the liver biopsy, the doctor announced: "Excellent news. As far as we can see, fatty infiltrates of the liver have not increased at all." Martin was not nearly as elated as the physician.

Martin's physician was treating a liver, not a whole person. Martin was depressed—not just sad, but suffering the clinical illness of depression. He had no motivation to work, no status, a low salary. He felt his efforts these past years had been a waste—"wasted" was exactly how he felt. Martin nevertheless did not recognize his disease as depression; he only knew that he felt "very, very tired."

Exhaustion is a common sign of depression. In fact, a depressed person's feeling of sadness can be masked so that fatigue and other physical symptoms may be the only indicators that something is seriously wrong. No wonder physicians sometimes search unrewardingly for a physical illness, tragically missing the correct diagnosis, a treatable depression.

Ned, an intense advertising executive, had both psychological *and* physical reasons for his fatigue. He came for a general physical and told me he was driving himself frantically to ward off a feeling of impending collapse. "At my core, I'm dog-tired. I could put the covers over my head for six months." He drank black coffee all day to fend off exhaustion.

Ned needed to analyze his living patterns. Stress was pervasive. His angry, competitive Type A life-style was particularly troubling in the light of his father's early heart disease and his own high blood pressure. Ned was preoccupied with "office politics and idiot clients." He couldn't obtain a decent night's sleep. Anxiety and depression loomed as prime suspects. But one more image imposed itself: that pot of coffee brewing in his office and the eight to ten cups he drank every day.

Far less coffee might upset the sleep of most individuals, but in Ned's case I suspected an even more significant problem. I instructed him to drink only decaffeinated coffee and to limit that to three times a day. Ned protested that he'd fold without caffeine. I advised him that his problem might be more than unrestorative sleep; his fatigue might be due to an addiction to coffee.

Ned stabilized after three harrowing days of caffeine withdrawal. One week later he felt more energetic and calmer than he had in years.

Ned had become caffeine-dependent. Initially, he had simply craved "sharpness" in his job performance and turned to coffee for a lift. However, as caffeine's stimulation wore off he sank back again. More coffee provided bursts of alertness, but also greater descents, as the addiction-withdrawal seesaw began to take hold. Other doctors had already counseled Ned about his high-stress life-style. However, he could begin work on the psychological issues that "drove him to drink" only after we had recognized and freed him from his physical addiction to caffeine.

Tracing the causes of fatigue involves fascinating investigations that should prove interesting as well as helpful. Certain causes of fatigue cross the cutting edge of nutrition research: how what we eat or fail to eat affects our energy. Others affect both the mind and body. These extremely important biological-psychological conditions include sleep disorders, chronic stress, and depression, conditions that are neither "all in the mind" nor "all in the body." One startling possibility is that fatigue in some individuals may be a kind of conditioned reflex, like that of Pavlov's dogs who learned to salivate at the sound of a bell. Several severely ill patients became almost completely normal when they learned to create more healthful conditionings with the aid of an unexpected therapy: medical hypnosis.

Many people who suffer fatigue need to give meticulous attention to any drugs they are taking—prescription drugs and over-the-counter medicines, to say nothing of such "recreational" drugs as alcohol or marijuana. Too often we overlook the critical role of medicines and drugs. Elements of the physical environment that affect our energy are also frequently not appreciated: air quality, noise volume, chemicals in food, weather changes, biological effects of light and color, computer display screens, and other environmental hazards in home and office. A complex interaction exists between the physical environment and our sense of well-being.

Of course, learning about fatigue will increase your understanding of your physical organs and how they interact. Many serious physical causes of fatigue can be misdiagnosed: adrenal gland insufficiency, hidden cancer of the bowel, subtle forms of heart disease, metabolic imbalances, nervous system disorders, and chronic viral or bacterial infections.

You may already be beginning to grasp that when it comes to fatigue even the very best doctors are still "practicing," still learning. Medicine remains an inexact art. We know a great deal, use incredible tools for diagnosis, and apply a wide array of effective treatments. However, our vast knowledge is fragmented. We need a perspective that can organize and connect the many forces that affect us. In this book I provide one such unified approach.

Chronic tiredness is a "final common pathway"—one symptom that can be the outcome of an extraordinary variety of causes. Fatigue is a sign that something in your complex body machine isn't right. Your job and your doctor's is to find the specific problem. My organized approach can help.

How to Make This Book Work For You

This book introduces you to many facts, but don't try to memorize them. It isn't necessary. You will nevertheless need an acquaintance with the facts to develop a sense for which causes of fatigue most likely affect you. Read each chapter at least once over lightly, *whether or not you expect it to be relevant to your problem.* My experience has shown that the answer often lies where we do not first expect it. Do not stop looking for causes when you meet the first disease or condition that is similar to yours.

Suppose, for example, your fatigue is accompanied by difficult breathing. Logically enough, you suspect a lung problem. However, shortness of breath should really suggest not just one but seven or eight prime suspects, including heart disease, metabolic imbalance, nerve-muscle deficiency, the hyperventilation syndrome and several others.

Don't attempt to decide which among your suspects is the real cause of your fatigue: that is your doctor's job. Your critical task is to focus your doctor's attention on the leading possibilities. With a sound list of prime suspects, diagnosis and treatment can proceed logically. Without such a list your efforts may flounder unless your problem is obvious or a rare lucky guess shows the way.

Be Informed and Be Assertive

Don't be shy about telling your doctor about your suspicions, even if they're based on nothing more than a feeling. A good doctor will not ridicule intuition. A patient's insights and observations are almost always real and meaningful, even when their explanation turns out to be different from what the doctor might first expect. Here is an example:

Sally Greer is a nurse whose cure started with an insight. She felt tired and irritable. Her eyes itched, her nose ran, and her sleep was troubled. She always felt worse in the winter and better in the spring. She had not thought much about this seasonal pattern until I asked her to read chapters from a draft of this book.

"That's it! Why didn't we think of it before?" She was reading about a newly recognized form of depression, a type that worsens each winter and improves every spring. Called Seasonal Affective Disorder (SAD), this form of depression may be triggered by deficient exposure to bright sunlight.

Mrs. Greer was correct. Her seasonal pattern was critical, but not for the reason she thought. After we reviewed her full history, we knew she wasn't really depressed—just tired and irritable. In fact, her history more accurately matched our description of indoor allergies and air pollution. Every November, Mrs. Greer closed her windows and "tightened" the insulation, causing the quality of air in her house to deteriorate. Decreased fresh air meant increased pollution from her husband's cigarette smoke, cat dander, and partially burned gas from the oven. This in turn caused her burning eyes, stuffy nose, restless sleep, and tired irritability.

Salvation came from cracking open her windows, putting a fresh air filter on the furnace, switching her gas oven to electric, banishing the cat from the bedroom, and sending her husband to a stop-smoking program.

Sally Greer became well because she had prepared her mind to recognize the significance of a critical clue, her seasonal pattern—*and* because she asserted herself to obtain my attention. My role as a doctor was also essential. I broadened her suspect list, evaluated each diagnosis and recommended treatment. She got well because we worked well together.

Communicating With Your Doctor

As you become better informed you will gain the additional skill of providing a clear medical history: a complete account of the most relevant matters in a form your physician can easily understand. The medical history is the most important ingredient for diagnostic success, even in this age of high technology. The patient who can provide a complete medical history is equipping the physician with information that is essential to diagnose what is likely to be wrong.

Many factors work against communicating a good history. High on the list are time, timidity, and disorganization.

Your doctor allocates ten or fifteen minutes to a routine office visit. This is fine for colds or blood pressure checks but is rarely enough for a problem as difficult and complicated as chronic fatigue. Don't try to crowd your diagnosis into one visit. Schedule a longer appointment or, better yet, a series.

Don't be timid, holding back important information. Follow the law of Wall Street: full disclosure. This is probably breached more often in the medical setting than in the world of finance. Because humans have a tendency to deny their worst fears, patients may neglect to tell doctors all their important symptoms.

For example, a man might visit a doctor because he feels tired all the time but not mention that he also feels a tightness in his chest when he climbs one flight of stairs. This symptom could be a sign of a serious heart or lung condition. He shouldn't coquettishly mention his weariness and leave it to omniscient Doc to discover the rest.

So be a complainer—you are really being a good information-giver. Complaining is better than stoically withholding facts, then reporting "None of my doctors were smart enough to find out what's wrong."

Getting Organized: The Why Am I Tired? Health History Form

Every doctor knows, theoretically, that valuable nuggets can be discovered in even the muddiest stream of talk. For example, a man telling about a conversation with a co-worker he couldn't hear may be informing the tuned-in doctor that he works in a noisy atmosphere—a common cause of fatigue. On the other hand, even the most attentive doctor can't pan all day for a rare nugget. You must therefore provide all the essentials, but do so succinctly. That is where good organization comes in.

The final but most important chapter of this book contains the *Why Am I Tired? Health History Form.* It will help you organize your history so the essential information stands out. Complete the form and share it with your doctor. It will save both of you time and help your doctor recognize which conditions should be prime suspects. As you work with the history form it should generate new questions and speculations. When this happens, reread the relevant chapters to deepen your understanding of the conditions that are prime suspects to be causes of your fatigue.

Of course, even telling a doctor "everything" won't identify everyone's problem. Some problems are unique to you; others may be too unusual or too new for your doctor to identify: the color in your office, peculiarities of your diet, the lighting on your video display terminal, a long-forgotten trauma of your childhood. Your health history form will highlight the topics about which you and your doctor need to learn more.

As you review the discussion of each cause of fatigue you will appreciate that each person's body, mind, and circumstances are unique. Your diagnosis and treatment must be tailored specifically to your needs. You deserve the best possible understanding of your problem. Combine knowledge from this book with the guidance of a good doctor and your desire to be well. That, together with a bit of luck, should lead to your feeling better in the weeks and months ahead.

Richard N. Podell, M.D.

Doctor, WHY *Am I So* TIRED?

PART 1

NUTRITION FACTS AND FALLACIES

CHAPTER

1

CAFFEINE

You are settled in a comfortable chair with a flavorful, aromatic cup of coffee, in your hand. The last thing you want to hear is that your favorite brew, the one you count on to combat fatigue, can cause a problem. For most people coffee is just what they'd like it to be—a tasty drink that revives the spirit. However, for people struggling with fatigue, coffee itself could be part of the problem.

Why is Coffee So Popular?

According to legend, the stimulating and invigorating effects of coffee were discovered by a goatherd named Kaldi in an ancient province in southwest Ethiopia. He observed the antics of his goats who had eaten the bright-red coffee berry, tried it himself, and proclaimed its delights throughout Africa and Arabia. Conservative Moslem priests decried coffee as intoxicating and, therefore, prohibited by the Koran.

Coffee attained popularity in the English-speaking world in the mid-1600s as London coffee houses became important social and political meeting places. In 1652, the first known advertisement for coffee declared that it "quickens the spirit and makes the heart lightsome." From the beginning, coffee's popularity derived from its pleasant stimulating effects on mind and body. These effects are the result of one main component of coffee: caffeine. Today about 80 percent of Americans drink coffee and other less potent caffeinated drinks.

Unfortunately, the uplifting effect for which we value caffeine has a less pleasant side: a letdown that can be so subtle you might not recognize caffeine's contribution to your fatigue.

Caffeine can cause fatigue in three major ways: by reducing the amount and quality of sleep; by overstimulating the mind and body; and by producing a kind of caffeine addiction. Tea, certain soft drinks, and some medications also have caffeine and can contribute to these problems. (Tables 1.1 and 1.2 give the caffeine content of foods and medicines.)

CAFFEINE AND SLEEP

If you are fatigued and have trouble falling asleep, staying asleep, or sleeping restfully, suspect that caffeine may be the cause when:

- You drink any caffeinated beverage within three hours of bedtime
- You drink the equivalent of five or more cups of coffee per day
- You observe that a small caffeine increase makes you restless, excited, super-alert, or nervous.

A single cup of coffee before bedtime will tend to increase the time it takes to fall asleep. Distracting physical discomfort, emotional upset, or noise can greatly amplify caffeine's activating effects. Caffeine also affects the quality of sleep, increasing the frequency of brief waking episodes throughout the night.

My experience indicates that reducing the overall intake of caffeinated beverages, particularly at dinner or later, often results in more restful sleep. Better sleep can alleviate the sense of fatigue that plagues you throughout the day.

Sensitivity to caffeine varies among people. Some individuals are

Table 1.1: APPROXIMATE CAFFEINE CONTENT OF BEVERAGES AND FOODS*

Source	*Food Quantity in ounces (oz.)*	*Caffeine Content in milligrams (mg)*
Chocolate, baking	1	35
Chocolate, bittersweet	1	20
Chocolate milk	8	8
Cocoa	6	5-10
Coffee, brewed	6	80-100
Coffee, decaffeinated	6	2-4
Coffee, instant	6	70-80
Milk chocolate bar	1	8
Soft drinks, caffeinated**	12	40-50
Tea	6	30-55

* You should strongly suspect caffeine-related problems when caffeine intake exceeds 500 mg per day.

** Caffeinated soft drinks include regular and diet colas as well as such noncola sodas as Mountain Dew, Orange Crush, Mellow Yellow, and Mr. Pibbs.

Table 1.2: APPROXIMATE CAFFEINE CONTENT OF COMMONLY USED MEDICINES

Medicine	*Milligrams (mg) Caffeine per unit dose*	*Medicine*	*Milligrams (mg) Caffeine per unit dose*
Dexatrim	200	Anacin Analgesic,	
Vivarin	200	Aspirin, A.P.C.,	
Cafergot	100	Bromo-Seltzer,	
Migralam	100	Capron, Cope,	
No-Doz	100	Darvon Compound,	approx. 30
Excedrin	65	Dolor, Midol,	
Pre-Mens	65	P-A-C Compound,	
Migral	50	Stanback Powder,	
Esgic	40	Trigesic, Vanquish	
Fiorinal	40		

fairly resistant to its stimulating effects; others seem to be extraordinarily sensitive. Without a caffeine-free trial period, you probably cannot tell if your customary caffeine intake is affecting your sleep.

CAFFEINE AND OVERSTIMULATION: THE STRESS-FATIGUE SEESAW

High doses of caffeine can wear you out by overstimulation, what I call the stress-fatigue seesaw. Remember one basic principle: what goes up must come down. A let-down is common after a period of overactivity. Fatigue induced by overstimulation also occurs with such diverse conditions as endocrine disorders (such as hyperthyroidism), medicines (epinephrine), and psychological distress (anxiety).

Initially, the upswing of the seesaw dominates. After drinking caffeine the heart's rate increases, as does its vigor of contraction. Blood pressure and breathing rate increase. The adrenal glands secrete their "fight/flight" hormones, adrenalin and cortisone. These activating effects are most noticeable with an abrupt increase in caffeine intake. With continued intake, tolerance develops, partially muting the body's stimulatory response.

For many coffee drinkers caffeine's stimulation is modest. Others become agitated or hyperalert. They may experience palpitation, difficulty concentrating, shortness of breath, sweating, headache, stomach upset, dizziness, or a feverish feeling. These upside hyperactive symptoms might later alternate with their opposites—downside symptoms of malaise, depression, and fatigue. Eventually burned-out lethargy and lack of motivation may be the dominant feelings.

Many caffeine victims realize that something is wrong. Others become so used to chronic overstimulation that they think it is normal for them: "I've always been a tense person." Only after they've been off coffee a while and feel the difference do these individuals truly understand how caffeine affects them.

Suspect that your fatigue may be caused by caffeine overstimulation if you drink the equivalent of five or more cups of coffee per day and you suffer symptoms of physical hyperstimulation or a sense of depletion. If cutting down on coffee makes you feel better, you have found a source of your problem.

CAFFEINE ADDICTION AND THE YOM KIPPUR EFFECT

In 1977, Rabbi Norman Lamm co-authored an article in the *New York State Journal of Medicine* that identified a problem for observant Jews who fast for twenty-four hours during the high holy day Yom Kippur. Rabbi Lamm described the lethargy, mental depression, drowsiness, inability to concentrate, fullness in the head, and severe headache that often occur during the all-day fast. He concluded that this syndrome was due to caffeine withdrawal and recommended gradually weaning off coffee during the week before Yom Kippur.

Caffeine dependence and chronic caffeine withdrawal are among the most common unrecognized causes of fatigue.

Caffeine withdrawal is easily recognized when coffee drinking suddenly stops. In one experiment high-intake coffee drinkers developed mild headache and tiredness within a few hours of their last cup. These symptoms increased dramatically during the first day. Runny nose, sweating, muscle aches, and leg pains began twelve to twenty-four hours after stopping. Decaffeinated coffee did not reduce symptoms, but regular coffee eliminated discomfort within two hours.

Many coffee drinkers are not aware of their dependence because they prevent withdrawal symptoms by drinking more coffee. They wake in the morning and can't quite get started until that first cup of coffee. They continue to drink throughout the day. As symptoms of sluggishness or vague headache appear, they reach for another cup. They say they feel fine, but closer questioning usually reveals sub-par functioning throughout much of the day.

Many heavy coffee drinkers doubt that coffee might be the cause of

Suspect that coffee dependence and withdrawal contribute to your tiredness if you drink five cups of regular coffee a day or the equivalent in other caffeinated foods or medicines and:

- You have frequent headaches or a haunting pressure in your head
- Past attempts to decrease caffeine produced drowsiness, or difficulty concentrating
- The idea of doing without coffee for even a day or two leaves you quaking.

their tiredness. "How could that be? Coffee is all that keeps me going." After a full withdrawal period of three to seven days, such persons are usually more alert and energetic than they've been in years. Their headaches are gone and they are calm and more relaxed.

If you can pass two full days without any caffeine and suffer no fatigue or headache, caffeine addiction is not your problem. Even so, you might still benefit by eliminating caffeine's sleep-disrupting and overstimulating effects.

Cut Back on Caffeine If You Suspect a Problem

First, discuss this with your doctor. He will help you decide whether the timing is right for you to withdraw from caffeine. For example, if you originally increased your caffeine to fight a depression, your doctor might advise you to postpone your withdrawal until the depression is treated.

If you doubt you are addicted to caffeine but suffer from poor sleep at night, you might continue your coffee but omit all caffeine after 4:00 P.M. Decaffeinated coffee might be all right since it contains only about 5 percent as much caffeine as regular coffee.

Most people deserve a completely caffeine-free holiday. A slow, tapered withdrawal (decreasing one cup a day until you are completely off caffeine) minimizes the intensity of withdrawal symptoms but drags out the time. Some people give up before they have the chance to discover how much better they can feel. I usually recommend a cold-turkey withdrawal followed by at least three weeks of abstinence. That way you quickly find out if caffeine addiction is a problem. Unfortunately, if you are addicted to caffeine, withdrawal symptoms can be distressing.

Set aside a few days when you don't have to function at your best. Even severely addicted people should feel okay in a week and terrific in two. During withdrawal I prefer to avoid all caffeine, including the small amount in decaffeinated coffee since a little caffeine might stimulate a craving for more.

If you do well you might reintroduce caffeine at a very low level after three weeks. However, be careful: "controlled drinking" can be tricky. It's usually better to continue withholding all caffeine for a full three months.

Once you are well, reflect on why you became overinvolved with caffeine. Was it simply its good taste and pleasant stimulation? Was it social pressure that might recur? Or did you feel you needed caffeine as a stimulant to get through the day? If so, caffeine may be only part of your problem. The reason you needed that lift might be just as important. Remember our friend, Ned, whose struggle with caffeine was described in the preface.

CHAPTER

2

SUGAR AND HYPOGLYCEMIA

Nearly everyone occasionally experiences sleepiness after a meal. Since we are not fortunate enough to live in a culture where it is common practice to take a siesta, drowsiness or fatigue often strikes just when we have to remain alert. Thus we know first-hand that food or drink can affect our energy.

One popular but controversial nutritional explanation for tiredness is *hypoglycemia* (low blood sugar). Anyone plagued with chronic tiredness will invariably encounter a friend (or a doctor) who will suggest that this is the cause. The hypoglycemia theory says that a sugary meal raises blood-sugar levels—triggering insulin, a critical hormone. Insulin drives blood sugar down, overshooting the mark. Thus blood-sugar levels three or four hours after eating are actually lower than before the last meal.

This rebound or reactive low blood sugar occurs in all of us and is perfectly normal. The difference, argue the hypoglycemia theorists, is that hypoglycemics release too much insulin, causing an excessive drop in blood sugar. This creates anxiety and hunger, which leads to eating again, further release of insulin, and an even greater fall in blood-sugar levels. Repeated metabolic turmoil creates multiple symptoms, including fatigue.

Consider the case of thirty-five-year-old Millie Robinson, who was always tired. She would have spells of nervousness, sweating, and dizziness. Her heart would race. She'd feel "spaced out," and have to struggle to think straight.

Mrs. Robinson's doctor told her she had fatigue and anxiety. "I know that," she said. "I want to know why." He offered a tranquilizer. She decided to pass.

She heard a radio nutritionist discuss hypoglycemia. The symptoms sounded exactly like hers . . . especially where her symptoms worsened just before mealtime. She could obtain relief from a doughnut, only to crash again later.

An endocrinologist told her "Hypoglycemia is just a fashionable excuse to explain away psychological neurosis. Doctors who believe in it are quacks." He ordered five hundred dollars' worth of blood and urine tests. Outcome: "Your endocrine glands are fine. Perhaps you should see a psychiatrist."

Mrs. Robinson's curiosity about hypoglycemia persisted since it was the first theory that took her complaints seriously. She read about treating it with a diet of frequent but modest meals. The diet excluded sugars and increased such protein foods as fish, poultry, meat, eggs, cheese, soy products, nuts, and beans. She gave it a try.

Three weeks later, she felt more energetic and calmer than she had in years. She began to see hope for a normal life. She returned to the endocrinologist, who said "Hypoglycemia? Ridiculous! I'm happy you feel better, but it's certainly not from your diet. It must be all in your head."

Most medical experts discount the hypoglycemia theory, but others consider it the primary cause of chronic fatigue. Hundreds of thousands of people swear by their antihypoglycemia diets. Are they fooling themselves? Or have the skeptics overlooked something important?

I believe the actual situation is this:

1. *The diet works.* About 40 percent of my patients whose history suggests a sugar-related problem improve after adopting an antihypoglycemia diet. Most continue to benefit for months or years. Thus I don't believe they are fooling themselves with a placebo effect (i.e., a treatment prescribed more for the mental relief of a patient than for its actual effect on his disorder).

2. *Why the diet works sometimes has nothing to do with sugar.* The diet excludes alcohol and coffee, which are themselves causes of chronic fatigue. The act of getting organized for the diet and of making the effort to help oneself may also be invigorating.

3. *Sugar restriction can help for reasons other than hypoglycemia.* Some people feel tired within an hour of eating a high-sugar meal. This is *not* hypoglycemia. True hypoglycemia should occur three to five hours later. People whose symptoms occur within an hour of eating are more likely to have too much tryptophan "on the brain."

Tryptophan is a sedating nutrient normally found in our blood. One effect of a high-sugar meal is to drive tryptophan from the blood into the brain. A high-protein meal does the opposite. This may be why many people feel tired on a junk-food diet and improve on a high-protein, low-sugar antihypoglycemia diet. Incidentally, tryptophan isn't always bad. In certain persons too little tryptophan may worsen depression.

Antihypoglycemia diets also offer superior general nutrition. Substituting vegetables and fruit for empty-calorie cookies and cakes increases vitamin and mineral intake. Indeed, processing sugar through the body's biochemical pathways actually removes vitamins and minerals from the body. If your vitamin or mineral nutrition is already marginal, a high-sugar diet could push you into deficiency.

A high-sugar, junk-food diet intensifies psychological wear and tear: those struggling to curb bad eating habits often suffer the fatiguing cycle of craving sweets, indulgence, and then remorse. Fortunately, your "sweet tooth" demands much less sugar once off sweets for a few weeks.

4. *You can have "hypoglycemia" and still have a normal blood sugar.* The most telling argument against the hypoglycemia theory is that most professed hypoglycemics actually have normal blood-sugar levels three to five hours after a meal. Then why do such people claim to feel better on the antihypoglycemia diet? Only recently have we begun to understand this paradox.

The explanation may be that "hypoglycemia" symptoms are usually not the result of low blood sugar itself but of the body's *hormonal reaction to prevent hypoglycemia from occurring.* In one careful study conducted at the University of Maryland School of Medicine, "hypoglycemics" had a massive discharge of adrenalin hormone at the precise moment their blood sugar reached the bottom of its fall. Adrenalin reverses falling blood sugar but is itself a trigger for anxiety, irritability, and—through them—fatigue.

5. *The traditional glucose tolerance test does more harm than good.* For generations the five-hour glucose tolerance test was considered the "gold standard" for diagnosing hypoglycemia. For this test one swallows a large amount of pure sugar; blood-sugar levels are measured over the next five hours. This test causes more confusion than clarification because many people who improve on the antihypoglycemia diet have relatively normal glucose tolerance tests. Others have an abnormal glucose tolerance result but absolutely no symptoms of hypoglycemia. Therefore, the five-hour glucose tolerance test should be abandoned for routine diagnosis.

Consider that sugar-related problems might contribute to your fatigue if:

- Medical and behavioral evaluation discloses no obvious cause
- Symptoms worsen within several days of increasing sugar or carbohydrate foods
- Symptoms worsen at a set time after eating, if your meal is delayed or if you overeat
- Symptoms improve with a low-sugar diet, a high protein-diet, or a high-fiber diet.

Suspect you do not have a sugar problem of importance if:

- You eat a strict antihypoglycemia diet for three weeks but don't improve
- You increase your sugar or junk-food intake for three weeks but don't get worse
- You learn that your health care practitioner diagnoses almost everyone as hypoglycemic.

Suspect you have a sugar problem plus other important problems if:

- You don't feel much better on an antihypoglycemia diet but do feel worse when you violate it
- You feel better on the antihypoglycemia diet but relapse within a few weeks or months despite remaining faithful to the diet
- Dietary sensitivities are becoming the overwhelming focus of your life.

Diagnosing Sugar-Related Disorders

If your symptoms suggest a sugar-related pattern, consider a three-week trial on an antihypoglycemia diet such as those described in Appendix 1. If you improve, your diet might be contributing to your fatigue. However, if you plan to change your diet for more than a few weeks, consult a physician or a registered dietitian who will work with your doctor. Speak frankly before your appointment. Avoid someone of the "sugar-is-good-for-you school." Such a person may not give adequate attention to your concern. Also avoid the "true believers" who think that diet should be the one and only issue in your life. They are likely to overlook other causes of fatigue whose symptoms can be almost identical to those of hypoglycemia.

If your doctor recommends a glucose tolerance test, be sure to note the timing of any symptoms that occur during the test. A nurse or technician should observe you to obtain an objective opinion of your reactions. Obtain a copy of the results to show future consultants.

Antihypoglycemia Diets

There are several antihypoglycemia diets: the original classic (low in carbohydrates and high in protein), the slightly sweeter modern version (low in sugar but high in complex carbohydrates and fiber), and the glycemic index (a new entry that is still being tested). Each calls for small but frequent meals, usually four to six servings a day. Each strictly limits caffeine and alcohol. Beyond that, there are important differences.

THE CLASSIC DIET

The original antihypoglycemia diet restricts sugar in all forms—cane, corn, beet, date, honey, and juice. It also limits other carbohydrate foods such as bread and potato. Protein foods are encouraged. Because of the long experience with it, this is my first choice for a three-week diagnostic trial.

The classic diet usually works well, but fatigue may get worse if the carbohydrate intake is too low. In addition, a low-carbohydrate diet can temporarily decrease one's tolerance for sugars if one overindulges. Taking some fat with each meal (vegetable oil, butter, cheese, fatty fish) tends to prevent this problem. The low-carbohydrate diet can be high in animal fat and thus not good for cholesterol-watchers. Substituting poultry, fish, and nuts for meat protein and cheese can control the cholesterol.

A high-protein diet is not recommended for people with certain kidney, liver, or metabolic disorders.

THE HIGH-COMPLEX CARBOHYDRATE, HIGH-FIBER, LOW-SUGAR DIET

The high-complex carbohydrate version is tastier and less restrictive than the classic diet. It is an excellent food plan for most of us, hypoglycemic or not. However you may be tempted to overload on such foods as whole wheat bread that actually convert rapidly into sugar. Some people feel better on the complex carbohydrate diet than with the classical low-carbohydrate approach. Others do better with the classic recipe. Examples of both diets can be found in Appendix 1.

THE GLYCEMIC INDEX REVOLUTION

In recent years scientists have measured the effects of specific foods on blood sugar using a new approach called the glycemic index. Some results are surprising. For example:

Table 2.1: GLYCEMIC INDEX (BLOOD-SUGAR RAISING ABILITY) OF COMMON FOODS*

Food	*Glycemic Index*	*Food*	*Glycemic Index*
BREADS		LEGUMES	
white bread	100	red lentils	43
whole wheat	100	kidney beans	51
sourdough rye	83	chickpeas	49
pumpernickel	80	baked beans	60
CEREAL GRAINS		lima beans	115
bulgur	65	peanuts	19
barley	31	FRUIT	
spaghetti	66	apple	53
rice	83	banana	79
BREAKFAST CEREALS		cherries	32
cornflakes	119	grapefruit	36
oatmeal (cooked)	85	grapes	66
shredded wheat	97	orange	67
VEGETABLES		orange juice	67
green peas	74	peach	40
carrots	133	pear	47
yam	74	plum	34
potato		raisins	93
boiled	81	SUGAR	
instant	116	sucrose (table sugar)	86
baked	135	DAIRY	
corn	87	ice cream	52
		milk	49
		yogurt	52

* The Glycemic Index measures the rise in blood sugar caused by a specific amount of each food compared to that caused by a reference food. In this case white bread has been chosen as the reference food and has been assigned a glycemic index of 100 percent. Adapted with permission from the *American Journal of Clinical Nutrition*, October 1985, p. 606.

White bread and whole wheat bread raise blood sugar equally.

Table sugar and ice cream cause blood sugar to rise less than do bread or potato.

Wheat eaten as spaghetti does not raise the blood sugar level as high as does wheat eaten as bread.

Foods that increase blood sugar least are soybeans, peanuts, kidney beans, lentils, and sweet fruit.

Table 2.1 compares the glycemic index of commonly eaten foods. A low number indicates that a food tends not to raise the blood-sugar level. In theory, such foods should not trigger an excessive insulin response and should be well tolerated by hypoglycemics. In this example white bread is arbitrarily given a glycemic index of 100.

Should traditional antihypoglycemia diets be altered to reflect the glycemic index of each food? Probably so, but we are not yet certain.

Risk of Being a Hypoglycemia Believer

I believe the hypoglycemia advocates are correct in concluding that a high-sugar diet can contribute to chronic fatigue, irritability, and other symptoms. However, the antihypoglycemia skeptics are also correct in charging that hypoglycemia believers sometimes go overboard.

Every physician has patients for whom hypoglycemia has become the central focus of life. Some of these individuals are using hypoglycemia as an excuse to avoid coming to terms with other serious physical or emotional problems.

Sometimes the doctor or nutritionist is at fault for fostering obsessive anxiety about hypoglycemia. However, often such persons were extremely vulnerable to anxiety before they learned about hypoglycemia. They are often intelligent, imaginative individuals who have the ability to create a web of fear out of a doctor's chance remark or a magazine article.

If you find yourself going overboard on the antihypoglycemia diet, remember that it is highly unlikely that all your problems occur because you are not strict enough with your diet. Don't withdraw into an ever-tightening circle of dietary restriction. Factors other than diet may contribute to your fatigue. Review the other chapters of this book with an open mind. Other causes of fatigue may also apply to your problem.

CHAPTER

3

VITAMINS AND MINERALS

Pam Roberts came to my office for a fourth opinion.

"I'm tired all the time. Is it because I don't eat right? I work full time and go to school at night. Regular eating is out of the question.

"I thought vitamins helped my energy, but now I'm not sure. My cousin is a nutrition professor. He said if I think vitamins help me, I must be imagining it. I asked another nutritionist for a second opinion. He sold me fifteen vitamins to take every day. I almost choked.

"My family doctor says that vitamins can't do any harm, but that a regular multivitamin is probably enough. I'm so confused I don't know what to think."

Pam is twenty-four, married, with no children yet. She has always been healthy, but for the past two years has found it hard to keep going. She eats at fast-food restaurants and snacks to keep going. She takes a birth control pill and a diuretic for fluid retention. Her physical examination was normal except for her weary appearance.

I explained that she is getting contradictory advice because there are three schools of thought about nutrition. The advice you receive depends almost entirely on who you ask. It's a catch-22 situation.

Pam's cousin, the professor, is from the conservative school. He believes that almost everyone can get enough vitamins and minerals from normal meals. He thinks that vitamin supplements to bolster energy are a complete waste of money. *Expensive urine* is his favorite phrase to describe what you get.

The second "nutritionist" is from the orthomolecular or megavitamin school. Megavitamin advocates teach that many people need high doses of vitamins to achieve optimal health. Nobel Prize winner Dr. Linus Pauling is the most prominent spokesman for the orthomolecular school.

Pam's family physician doesn't claim to know much about nutrition. However, he believes that improper eating habits are unhealthy and that a multivitamin might help. He reflects the influence of what I call the progressive school. They don't believe in megavitamins but do believe that nutritional deficiencies are fairly common. This is my bias as well.

Pam saw my registered dietitian for an analysis of her diet. The dietitian concluded that Pam's eating was lopsided, favoring so called empty calories—highly processed sugars that are poor in vitamins and minerals. She was weak on vegetables and essential vegetable oils. Her birth control pill was another concern because it depletes the body of vitamin C, folic acid, and vitamin B_6. Her "water pill" or diuretic depletes potassium and magnesium.

I ordered tests for blood vitamin and mineral levels. Pam's result was below normal for Vitamin B_1 (thiamine), the most critical vitamin for metabolizing sugar. She was also low in folic acid, vitamin C, iron, and borderline in the minerals zinc, potassium, and magnesium. Severe deficiency of any one of these nutrients could certainly cause fatigue.

The dietitian taught Pam how to obtain a more balanced diet despite her tough schedule. For insurance we added a broad-spectrum vitamin/mineral supplement containing roughly one RDA (recommended dietary allowance) of most vitamins and minerals. We switched her diuretic to one that does not waste potassium or magnesium. We urged careful scheduling and pacing so she would have time for nutrition and also time for herself.

Pam's energy increased during the next few months. With a few ups and downs, she has stayed well for three years. Of course, we don't know for sure whether her improvement was from better nutrition. Our life-style counseling probably helped. My guess is that both were important.

Are Nutritional Deficiencies Common?

Individuals with nutrition profiles like Pam's are not rare. Federal statistics indicate that millions of Americans do not eat the recommended daily allowance for one or more major vitamins or minerals. At especially high risk are the elderly, the poor, teenagers, people on the go, small children, hospital in-patients, nursing-home residents, those with chronic illness, people taking certain medicines, crash dieters, food faddists, and heavy drinkers of alcohol.

Between 20 percent and 50 percent of older Americans eat less than two-thirds of the recommended dietary allowance for one or more important vitamins. Their average intake of zinc is less than 70 percent of the RDA. Fifteen percent eat less than half the RDA of magnesium. Thirty percent of older women eat less than half the recommended amount of calcium.

The conservative school counsels "Don't worry" and points out, correctly, that RDAs are set to provide a large margin of safety. Minor deficiencies, they claim, should not make you tired.

Despite such reassurances, many nutritionists are concerned that "minor" deficiencies do matter. Our body requires every vitamin and mineral for its biochemical systems to work optimally. At what point does deficiency reduce the effectiveness of these reactions? Unfortunately, nutrition scientists haven't studied this question thoroughly. Logic suggests that even slight deficiencies could affect us and should be corrected when possible.

A BRIEF SURVEY OF VITAMINS AND MINERALS

Vitamin B_1 (thiamine). Dr. Derrick Lonsdale of the Cleveland Clinic found mild vitamin B_1 deficiency among many teenagers who complained of fatigue and irritability. Most improved when they took vitamin B_1 supplements.

Severe vitamin B_1 deficiency can cause personality changes, including depression and psychosis, as well as permanent damage to the nervous system. Increased need for Vitamin B_1 occurs with high-carbohydrate diets, high alcohol consumption, pregnancy, lactation, and illness.

Sources of vitamin B_1 include whole grains, brewer's yeast, peanuts, brown rice, legumes (peas and beans), nuts, egg yolk, organ meats, fish, red meat, poultry, and fresh vegetables.

Vitamin B_3 (niacin, niacinamide, nicotinic acid). Fatigue is an early sign of vitamin B_3 deficiency. Advanced deficiency causes diarrhea, depression, and skin problems. Before vitamin supplementation was common, perhaps half the state mental hospital beds in some Southern states were occupied by unrecognized victims of pellagra, a vitamin B_3 deficiency disease.

Good sources of vitamin B_3 include milk, beef, liver, yeast, cheese, leafy green vegetables, peanuts, poultry, fish. The amino acid tryptophan is also a source of vitamin B_3 activity. Niacin vitamin supplements can cause a sudden flush, that some find disturbing. In high doses niacin serves as a drug for lowering cholesterol. However, high doses can cause liver damage, activate ulcers, and worsen diabetes.

Vitamin B_6 (pyridoxine). Vitamin B_6 deficiency can cause fatigue, nerve damage, seizure disorders, and anemia. Several important drugs bring out vitamin B_6 deficiency: birth control pills, the antituberculosis drug Isoniazid (INH), and the high blood pressure medicine Apresoline (hydralazine). Some women who develop depression while taking birth control pills may be helped by vitamin B_6 supplements.

Good nutritional sources of B_6 include wheat germ, liver, nuts, milk, eggs, beef, poultry, soy flour, banana, avocado, cabbage, cauliflower, and dried fruit. Vitamin B_6 megadoses can cause nerve damage with numbness and tingling. Beware of supplements with 500 mg a day or more. The RDA for B_6 is only 2 mg for adults.

Vitamin B_{12}. B_{12} shots for fatigue are a hallowed tradition. Most experts believe B_{12} shots "work" because of a placebo effect: that is, because the recipients expect the shot will help. However, some people do have a measurable vitamin B_{12} deficiency. A few rare individuals require larger-than-expected amounts of B_{12} for their enzymes to work well.

Strict vegetarians—who eat no meat, dairy, fish, or eggs—are at risk for B_{12} deficiency, since B_{12} is absent in vegetable foods. Alcoholics and people with disease of the stomach or intestine may have trouble absorbing vitamin B_{12}. Pernicious anemia is a form of vitamin B_{12} deficiency that results from inadequate B_{12} absorption.

Liver and kidney are excellent sources. Moderate amounts of B_{12} occur in meats, fish, eggs, and fermented cheese. Contrary to popular belief, for most people vitamin B_{12} shots provide no advantage over B_{12} in food or in pill form.

Folic Acid. Folic acid deficiency is relatively common. Severe deficiency can lead to fatigue, depression, and anemia. Alcohol, birth control pills, certain cancer chemotherapy drugs, and Dilantin—an antiepilepsy medicine—deplete or antagonize folic acid. A University of Alabama study suggests that women on birth control pills may develop abnormal, precancerous Pap smears because of the pill's interference with folic acid nutrition. Folic acid supplements tend to correct this.

Excellent sources include deep-green leafy vegetables, carrots, yeast, liver, egg yolk, cantaloupes, apricots, pumpkins, avocados, beans, and whole wheat. Folic acid supplementation can antagonize the action of vitamin B_{12}. People taking folic acid should have their vitamin B_{12} levels checked first. Extremely large doses of folic acid can disturb brain-wave patterns.

Vitamin A. Although vitamin A deficiency is rampant in much of the world, most Americans get more vitamin A than they need. Deficiency signs include dry eyes, dry skin, and night blindness. Mild vitamin A deficiency might increase vulnerability to cancer. Manufacturers add Vitamin A as a supplement to whole milk. Natural sources include green and yellow vegetables, liver, and eggs.

Vitamin A overdose can cause fatigue, headache, dry skin, loss of hair, brittle nails, and vague abdominal complaints. Because vitamin A is stored in the liver and in fatty tissue it tends to accumulate. Therefore most people should not need a supplement higher than the RDA, or about 5000 International Units (IU). Carotene, a nutrient related to vitamin A, is probably as effective but is less likely to be toxic. Indeed, there is strong evidence that carotene and related compounds in fruit and vegetables might diminish the risk of certain forms of cancer. Carotene is also sold as a supplement.

Vitamin C. Severe vitamin C deficiency causes tiredness, weakness, depression, loss of appetite, and vague pains many months before the characteristic bruises of scurvy appear. Unfortunately, we do not know what harm may occur from mild vitamin C deficiency.

Vitamin C is plentiful in citrus fruit, berries, green and leafy vegetables, tomatoes, cauliflower, potato, and sweet potato. The RDA for adults is 40 to 60 milligrams. However, one can make a good argument for supplementing to levels several times this amount.

Potassium. Potassium deficiency causes fatigue, muscle weakness, heartbeat irregularities, and difficulty concentrating. The most common cause is the potassium-wasting effect of diuretic pills. Alcoholism also exacerbates potassium loss. Mild potassium deficiency sometimes exists despite normal blood-potassium levels.

Potassium can be found in citrus fruit, all green leafy vegetables, watercress, banana, potato, dried fruit, and sunflower seeds. The best treatment for low potassium is prevention. Your doctor can switch you to a diuretic that does not waste potassium, prescribe potassium supplement tablets, or measure your blood-potassium level regularly to spot a downward trend.

Magnesium. Magnesium deficiency causes fatigue, personality changes, muscular irritability, and heartbeat irregularities. Low magnesium can result from diuretics, high alcohol intake, poor gastrointestinal absorption, and certain anticancer and antifungal medicines.

Good food sources include nuts, seeds, and green vegetables. In hard-water areas drinking water contains significant magnesium. However, one can have a normal blood-magnesium level and still be magnesium-depleted.

Zinc. Mild zinc deficiency may depress certain immune cell functions, especially in the elderly. It can also retard growth in adolescents and delay sexual maturity. Modest zinc deprivation of pregnant monkeys leads to lethargy, apathy, and decreased activity in their infants. Humans at high risk for zinc deficiency include diabetics, sickle cell anemia victims, the elderly, low-income people, and alcoholics.

Food sources include seafood, organ meats, muscle meat, mushrooms, sunflower seeds, pumpkin seeds, brewer's yeast, and soybean.

Iron. Iron deficiency is extremely common among menstruating women. Recent research suggests that iron deficiency even without anemia might cause fatigue and difficulty concentrating. This is important because, even with decent nutrition, it is difficult to eat enough iron to keep up with menstrual loss. That is why many menstruating women should take an iron supplement.

Food sources include liver and other organ meats, fish, poultry, eggs, cherry juice, green leafy vegetables, dried fruit, shellfish, and nuts.

Men and nonmenstruating women rarely develop iron deficiency caused by poor nutrition. Subtle blood loss from the gastrointestinal tract is a more common reason for iron deficiency among these groups. If bleeding is the problem iron supplements might be harmful, since they could mask the early symptoms of an important disease process.

Calcium. Physicians are debating the importance of calcium deficiency as a cause both of the bone disease osteoporosis and of high blood pressure. High and low blood-calcium levels both cause fatigue. The reason is usually not malnutrition but a breakdown in the body's ability to regulate calcium's metabolism. If blood-calcium levels are abnormal it is imperative to find the cause.

Except among those with certain metabolic, liver, or kidney diseases, there should be almost no risk of serious side effects from taking vitamin/mineral supplements at about 100 percent of the RDA. Many might benefit. It is wise, therefore, to err on the side of nutritional adequacy by the intelligent use of supplements, even if you risk getting a bit more than the minimum nutrition you need. The price is right too. Standard supplements can supply about 100 percent of the RDA for about twelve cents a day. Appendix 3 lists the recommended dietary allowances for most vitamins and minerals.

Massive Vitamin Doses

If you feel better when you increase your sleep time from seven hours to eight, will you feel even better by trying for nine or ten? Usually not. Unfortunately, some individuals make this mistake with their vitamins and minerals—if a little is good, more must be better.

Orthomolecular nutritionists believe many ills result because the body's biochemistry does not function optimally. They contend that people often have defects in enzymes, biochemical elements essential to metabolism. The orthomolecular school believes that high levels of vitamins and minerals can correct enzyme defects, which then leads to better health. Thus an orthomolecular nutritionist might view fatigue as a problem of enzyme metabolism and hope to improve metabolism by prescribing very large doses (megadoses) of nutritional supplements, typically fifty to a hundred times the RDA.

The basic theory of the orthomolecular school is correct under certain circumstances. Dozens of diseases result from subtle biochemical defects, which can be corrected with megadose nutrients. But almost all these diseases are extremely rare. *None* of our most common diseases, including the known causes of fatigue, has been shown to improve with megavitamins.

Certain megadose treatments are intriguing and might someday prove valuable. However, as the evidence stands today, I cannot recommend orthomolecular treatments except in unusual circumstances.

Unfortunately, megadose nutritional treatments can sometimes be dangerous. Overdose of the fat-soluble vitamins A and D can cause fatigue and more serious problems. Vitamin B_6 megadoses cause nerve damage. Mineral supplements can be toxic even at relatively low multiples of the RDA. Amino acid supplements have a special potential for overdose toxicity.

How to Tell if You Need More Vitamins and Minerals

Blood-vitamin levels can be measured directly. Although not perfect, blood-vitamin levels provide a reasonable measure of your nutritional status.

Blood levels of minerals such as potassium, magnesium, iron, calcium, and zinc can also be measured. Normal blood levels do not guarantee adequate nutrition, but low levels usually are significant. Hair analysis may be a useful screen for exposure to toxic minerals such as lead, cadmium, mercury, or arsenic but, despite claims to the contrary, hair analysis is not yet reliable for most nutritional purposes.

How to Choose a Vitamin/Mineral Supplement

If you're always tired and can't find out why, the best insurance against vitamin/mineral deficiency is a supplement that provides about one RDA of each vitamin and mineral. (The content of each nutrient should be on the label.) This amount, together with nutrients from your diet, is usually enough. Except in rare circumstances, it should be totally safe.

Unfortunately, most popular supplements provide more B vitamins than you need, but only scant amounts of most minerals. One that comes close to sensible amounts is (appropriately) called Insurance Formula and is made by the Bronson Company. Other fairly well-balanced supplements include Centrum (Lederle), High Potency Vitalizer (Taylor), Mega Plus (Westpro), One a Meal (Rich Life), One-a-Day Plus Minerals (Miles), RDA (Schiff), and Theragran M (Squibb). Mineral supplements sometimes cause stomach upset. If so, a plain multivitamin should be your alternative.

Of course, you can usually obtain all the nutrition you need from your food, if you teach yourself how and continue to work at it.

Who Can Help You Decide Whether Your Nutrition Affects Your Fatigue

There is no one "correct" viewpoint on most nutritional problems, including the link between fatigue and what you eat. In a very real sense, *you* are the doctor, because your choice of advisor and the school of thought that he or she adheres to will largely determine the advice you will get. There is no way around it. An orthomolecular physician will probably recommend orthomolecular treatment. A conservative nutritionist will recommend a sound diet but assume your fatigue is not related. A progressive middler will hedge, but probably offer low-dose nutritional supplements and dietary advice.

CHAPTER

4

FOOD ALLERGY AND FATIGUE

Is food allergy the reason you are tired? Like so many nutrition theories, this one is controversial. The leading supporters of a food-allergy approach are nonmainstream physicians known as clinical ecologists. They believe that everyday foods such as milk, wheat, eggs, or yeast can trigger health problems including fatigue, headache, bowel irritability, skin conditions, depression, and anxiety.

Clinical ecologists believe reactions to frequently eaten foods are often unnoticed because foods remain in our system for forty-eight hours or more after eating. This obscures the relationship between when you eat and when you have symptoms. Until recently, very few prominent physicians thought the food-allergy approach made sense. But several recent studies support the theory that food reactions account for some cases of eczema, migraine headache, hives, and irritable bowel syndrome. There is even one extremely well-researched case of rheumatoid arthritis swelling triggered by milk. Could fatigue be another condition in which food allergy participates? Perhaps not often, but I have seen instances where this seems likely.

I recall a young psychologist who could not stay awake. She told me that she was fine until noon, but then began to fade out. If she didn't eat until dinner she remained well until then. Wheat and milk were the two foods she ate every day for lunch and dinner, but rarely for breakfast. Eliminating these eliminated her problem. No problem occurred when she resumed drinking milk, but reintroducing wheat reproduced all her symptoms.

The Food-Allergy Controversy: State of the Science

Although some individuals sincerely believe their fatigue regularly follows eating one or more specific foods, no one has evaluated these claims in a carefully controlled scientific study. Until recently there were few decent studies of the effects of food on any symptoms. Fortunately, we are now beginning to see some solid evaluations, and these seem to suggest that there may be some value to the food-allergy theory as it relates to several conditions.

Eczema. Probably the most important current work on food allergy is that of Dr. Hugh Sampson, formerly of Duke and now of Johns Hopkins. Dr. Sampson studied children who have eczema—a skin disease characterized by a rash and itching. Many parents of children with eczema believe that their child's skin condition gets worse after eating certain foods. Most physicians discount this belief as innaccurate, wishful thinking, or mere coincidence.

Sampson applied meticulous research methods to study a large group of children with severe eczema. Central to his method is the fact that he observed children who were fed their suspect food after it had been hidden in an opaque capsule. In that way neither the child nor the observers knew when the children had eaten the suspect food and when they had taken a harmless placebo. This avoids the bias of anticipating results typical of many earlier studies. Sampson questioned each child about symptoms after each feeding, observed skin changes, and also measured the blood level of histamine, a chemical released during allergic reactions.

Sampson's results forcefully contradict the traditional skepticism. Although there were many instances in which suspect foods did not trigger reactions, about half the children did develop a reaction after eating a suspect food but not after a placebo. Of these, about 90 percent complained of itching and developed a rash. However, many also evolved nasal stuffiness, intestinal upset, and/or asthma. Blood-histamine levels often increased, confirming the allergic nature of the reactions. Little change occurred after eating a placebo.

Many dermatologists remain skeptical. However, most allergists now accept that food allergy plays an important role in some children with eczema.

Migraine headache. Serious study of the relationship between foods and migraine is under way. Dr. Lyndon Mansfield at Texas Tech University in El Paso studied forty-three adults with recurrent migraine headaches. Sixteen had positive skin tests to one or more foods. Eleven of these sixteen improved after a change in diet to eliminate potential food allergens. Seven individuals agreed to a double blind study in which they would eat either the "allergic" food or a placebo. Five developed migraine eating a suspect food. Of these three showed a rise in blood histamine. None reacted after the placebo.

Many, but not all, allergists now believe that food allergy plays a role in at least some cases of migraine in adults.

Even more dramatic results were found among children with frequent migraine headache by doctors at London's Hospital for Sick Children. Eighty-eight children volunteered for a strict elimination diet. Seventy-eight improved to the point at which they rarely required medicines. Foods were reintroduced one at a time to discover potential headache triggers. Possible reactions were found to an average of 2.7 foods or food additives per person.

To decide whether these reactions were coincidental or placebo effects, forty children then entered a double blind study. They ate their suspect food allergens for a week disguised in a porridge so they did not know whether they were eating that food or a placebo. Twenty-eight of theforty developed headache while eating their suspect food. Only two had headaches while eating the placebo. In contrast to Mansfield's study, where allergy skin tests had identified most reacting foods, the London group found that most foods that seemed to trigger headache were not "allergies" in the usual sense. Traditional skin and blood allergy tests were negative. If the London group is correct, much of the problem in childhood migraine is a form of sensitivity to foods distinct from classical allergy. This could be a critical insight, because such "non-allergic" food sensitivities will always be missed in an allergy examination that relies on traditional skin or blood tests.

Unfortunately, no one has repeated the London study. Therefore, migraine specialists do not accept its conclusion that most children with frequent migraine suffer mainly from food sensitivity. Physicians should be wary of accepting any conclusion based on a single study, even one that appears as well-designed as this one. Therefore, until another research group takes on the time-consuming task of reproducing the London study's results, we will not know for sure whether food sensitivity is an important factor in this distressing disease.

The Allergic Irritability Syndrome. Recently, a committee of the American College of Allergy, a leading professional organization of allergists, encouraged allergists to accept the existence of an allergic irritability syndrome: symptoms of emotional irritability and temper tantrums that sometimes occur as a complication of allergy. Fatigue is frequently part of this syndrome. Indeed, it was previously recognized by many allergists under the label of *allergic tension fatigue syndrome.* Although not focused on food allergy per se, this position statement supports previous reports that allergy can affect mental and emotional well-being.

Irritable-Bowel Syndrome. Irritable bowel—intermittent diarrhea, constipation, cramps, or gas—affects a quarter or more of American adults. A high proportion of its victims also complain of fatigue. Researchers in the department of immunology at Cambridge University found in a double blind study that fourteen of twenty-one irritable-bowel patients developed symptoms after eating specific foods. Doctors at the University of Manchester also found confirmed food reactions, but in a lower proportion—three out of twenty-seven patients. Thus, food reactions can be important, but we do not know if this applies to only a few irritable-bowel patients or to the majority.

My practice's experience is that about a fourth of irritable-bowel patients discover important food sensitivities and that these are mostly not "allergies," since traditional allergy testing is negative. Sometimes, but not always, when the bowel improves after changing the diet, the accompanying fatigue also improves.

Rheumatoid Arthritis. Possibly the most surprising food allergy result is from Dr. Richard Panush at the University of Florida College of Medicine in Gainesville. Dr. Panush set out to disprove the effect of a popular antiarthritis diet. He showed that the diet in question did not work but noticed that a few patients did seem to get worse after they ate certain foods. He placed one subject who claimed reactions to milk on a medical school research ward. He freeze-dried milk, placed the powder in an opaque capsule, and repeatedly fed her either milk or placebo. Her arthritis symptoms and joint swelling flared each time after milk but never after placebo. The usual allergy antibody, known as the IgE antibody, was negative to milk, but a less common allergy antibody called IgG did react. Food allergy as a cause of arthritis is certainly not common, but Dr. Panush's research indicates that it can occur.

Most reports about food allergy and food sensitivity have been based on hearsay. Fortunately, respected scientists are now applying good scientific method to evaluate these reports. Although food sensitivity probably affects a minority of people, it is a genuine phenomenon. Probably it is more common and important than we used to believe.

If Not a Food Allergy, What Is It?

One problem is that in looking for traditional forms of allergy we may have overlooked other types of reactions to food. A fascinating example comes from Boston's Children's Hospital. Harvard Medical School researchers studied twelve children with a rare condition called eosinophilic gastroenteropathy. In this disease inflammatory cells called eosinophiles infiltrate the stomach or intestines, causing diarrhea, malabsorption, and other serious symptoms. Six children had definite food allergy: they had positive skin tests and became worse after that food (usually milk). However, eliminating their allergic foods had little effect on the severity of their illness. Thus, their food allergy, although genuine, was not the fundamental cause of their disease.

In contrast, the other six children got completely well when cow's milk was withdrawn from the diet. Ironically, these milk-sensitive children were not allergic in the traditional sense. Their skin and blood allergy tests for milk were negative. They had also been drinking milk without anyone's noting its effect on their symptoms. These children do not have food allergy, but their food sensitivity was critical to their illness.

There is clearly more to this field than we previously thought. Allergy, as we have usually defined it, is only part of the story. Food sensitivity may be as important or more so. However, since there are no skin or blood tests for most forms of food sensitivity, a proper evaluation requires confirming suspicions using an elimination diet.

When to Suspect Food Allergy or Sensitivity

These are clues that might indicate a food problem:

- Reacting adversely to a specific food on at least three occasions.
- A strong allergy to inhalant allergens such as dust, mold, pollen, or animal dander.
- A strong family history of allergies or food reactions.

- Chronic bowel complaints such as gas, cramps, diarrhea, constipation—the irritable-bowel syndrome.
- Multiple symptoms that are not well explained by physical illness or psychological factors.
- Unusual adverse reactions to chemical smells such as perfume, auto exhaust, household cleaners, new fabrics, or newsprint.

The last two clues are particularly intriguing.

Many people who are diagnosed as having food allergies also suffer from a broad spectrum of symptoms: fatigue, headaches, backache, depression, stomach upset. It is as if their entire body were involved in the illness. We do not understand why this occurs.

Many, but not all, food-allergy patients also develop symptoms after exposure to common chemical smells. A similar sensitivity is fairly common among people with migraine headache, asthma sufferers, and some pregnant women. We discuss a dramatic case of a patient with food and chemical sensitivity in Chapter 13.

How to Diagnose Food Allergy

To the conventional allergist, allergy means an unusual reaction caused by the IgE antibody, the antibody that causes redness and swelling in a standard allergy skin test. By this definition, much that is diagnosed as food allergy should really be called nonallergic sensitivity, since the IgE antibody is often not involved.

Conventional allergies can be detected by standard skin tests or by a special IgE blood test called a RAST (Radioallergosorbent Test). Unfortunately there is no simple, accurate test for nonallergic sensitivity. The best is an old-fashioned, low-technology one: the elimination diet.

HOW TO DO AN ELIMINATION DIET

The most accurate way to test for food sensitivities is to live for several days or weeks eating only a predigested liquid formula diet called Vivonex. Vivonex contains no food antigens, so theoretically it cannot cause allergic reactions. (I have seen rare exceptions.) It is nutritionally well balanced and can be the sole source of nutrition for several weeks or longer. However, Vivonex is fairly expensive and far from delicious. I have used it successfully, but it is not a picnic.

The oligoantigenic (literally: few-antigen) diet is more practical. This diet restricts you to a short list of foods that you previously ate once weekly or less, that you enjoy, and that do not seem to cause problems.

An oligoantigenic diet might include one meat (perhaps lamb or turkey), one or two starches (rice, sweet potato, or oatmeal), a fruit (such as pear), a vegetable (green beans, broccoli), a cooking oil (safflower, olive), salt, water, and perhaps a multivitamin/mineral supplement.

It is important to eat and drink large amounts since *undereating can cause complications.* If there is no improvement after two weeks or so, food sensitivity is probably not causing your symptoms. If you do improve, food sensitivity might be the reason.

If you improve on the elimination diet, reintroduce one or two foods at a time to see which bring back your symptoms. Repeat them for two successive meals. Those that provoke no reaction are safe and can return to the diet. Suspicious foods are set aside, to be tried again later. If you suspect only a few foods, eliminate these. Then reintroduce them to see their effect.

Ideally, to reduce the placebo effect, suspect foods should be disguised in opaque capsules or blended into a porridge. However, creating workable disguises is expensive and time-consuming. (An accomplice can give you a strong-tasting blenderized shake or mash that disguises the food's taste.) A good compromise is to reintroduce each food openly at first, concocting blind challenges later for only those foods that seem to cause problems.

Plan your elimination diet with your doctor. Such diets are relatively safe, but not completely so. Undereating and dehydration can be a problem. The effect of medicines such as the antidepressant Lithium can be amplified, creating the equivalent of an overdose. Severe asthma, hives, or allergic shock can occur (although rarely) when highly allergic foods are reintroduced.

A modification of the elimination diet is to omit only those foods you already suspect cause you problems or that are commonly reported as causes of food sensitivity. Liberalizing the elimination diet will cause you to miss a few genuine food problems, but probably not many. Most food-allergy studies find more than two-thirds of the reactions are from milk, egg, peanut, wheat, soy products, chicken, yeast, fish, corn, and orange. In small children especially, milk and eggs together account for the largest proportion. Whether food colorings or preservatives are important remains controversial. I prefer to keep them away during the elimination diet study.

For example, you might try the Cave Man or Stone Age Diet, a favorite with many old-time food allergists. This diet permits any foods that one imagines were available to primitive man before the dawn of agriculture. Thus, you are permitted meat, poultry, fish, nuts, seeds, fruit, and vegetables. You omit all grains (wheat, rice, corn, and so on), sugar, milk products (including cheese), yeast or fermented products (including alcohol), eggs, and any foods with preservatives, colors, or flavors added.

Give yourself a week or two to get used to the Cave Man Diet. It can be nutritionally sound and fully satisfying, but it forgoes many modern conveniences. Judge how you feel in the second or third week. Of course improvement while on the Cave Man Diet might be coincidental. Or your problem might be nutritional but not related to specific food sensitivity. For example, the Cave Man Diet is not much different from the classic antihypoglycemia diet or the antiyeast diet we will meet in Chapter 5.

Another form of elimination diet preferred by many clinical ecologists is the rotary diversified or rotation diet. This diet does not allow you to eat the same food a second time until after several days have elapsed. The rotation diet was developed on the principle that you are more likely to recognize reactions to a food eaten intermittently than to the same food when eaten every day. Food-allergy diagnosis with the rotation diet provides only one or two foods at each meal and repeats the same food only once every four days. For example, if you have egg for breakfast on Monday (day 1), you have no more egg products again until Friday (day 5). If you are sensitive to eggs you should recognize the pattern because your symptoms should occur with some regularity on the days you eat egg. Your initial choices are confined to foods that are unlikely to cause problems. After a pattern of "safe" foods is established, new foods are tested by adding them to the rotation. Appendix 2 provides two sample four-day rotation diets that can be used for diagnosis of food allergy and food sensitivity under the supervision of a physician.

Food-Allergy Terrors: The Downside of Food Allergy

Food-allergy terrors are symptoms caused by anticipation or fear. Their occurrence may be the most important risk of becoming involved in a search for food allergies.

Mrs. Kaye had always been a worrier. About three months before seeing me she had noticed exhaustion accompanied by headaches, nervousness, and stomach cramps after eating milk and sugar. Then her "allergies" spread to include wheat, eggs, yeast, beef, and soy products. She was losing weight and was in a panic. Her chronic worry about eating led to a sense of worn-out fatigue.

She had been under stress for quite a few years, so she joined our stress management program. We teach relaxation by imagining calm situations, relaxing muscles, controlling breathing, and self-hypnosis to trigger the relaxation response whenever stressful situations occur. For Mrs. Kaye we added an additional self-hypnosis suggestion—she would imagine herself being able to eat her "allergic" foods without problems. Within a month she had almost completely recovered.

Most likely Mrs. Kaye's problem began with a genuine food reaction. Then her anxiety caused her to focus extra attention on small changes in her body each time she ate. Symptoms she would ordinarily overlook would then trigger panic: "There it goes again." Already hypervigilant by nature, each "reaction" would prime her for the next. By reversing these events, the hypnotic suggestion led to her "cure."

It can be extraordinarily difficult to distinguish between a genuine food sensitivity and one created by fear.

CYTOTOXIC BLOOD TESTING FOR FOOD ALLERGIES

Widely promoted, the "cytotoxic" blood test has become an allergist's nightmare. Its results are wrong more often than they are right. Make a point of avoiding it.

Choosing a Consultant

If your symptoms fit those of the food-allergy profile, you have already explored more conventional approaches, and you recognize that the food-allergy approach remains controversial, you might consider discussing your concerns with a conventional allergist or a clinical ecologist.

Well-trained allergists are usually members of the American Academy of Allergy and Immunology or of the American College of Allergists. They tend to be conservative, but many are willing to work with elimination diets. If you seek a more aggressive (although controversial) approach consult a member of the American Academy of Environmental Medicine, the organization to which most clinical ecologists belong.

Discuss your plans with your personal physician. He or she may not be an expert on allergy or nutrition but should be an expert on you. Your doctor can help you be realistic as you navigate this still murky area.

CHAPTER

5

THE CANDIDA YEAST THEORY

The Candida Yeast Theory of Fatigue: Misleading Fad or Medical Breakthrough?

If you answer yes to seven or more of these questions, your symptoms are "almost certainly" related to a candida yeast problem, according to allergist Dr. William G. Crook*:

Do you experience fatigue, depression, poor memory, or nervous tension?

Do you crave sugar, breads, or alcoholic beverages?

Have you ever taken antibiotics on a frequent basis?

Do you have recurrent digestive problems?

Are you bothered by hives, psoriasis, or other chronic skin rashes?

Have you ever taken birth control pills?

Have you ever been troubled by premenstrual tension, abdominal pain, menstrual problems, vaginitis, or loss of sexual interest?

Does exposure to tobacco, perfume, pesticides, household cleansers, or other chemical odors provoke moderate to severe symptoms?

Are you bothered by headaches, poor coordination, or pains in your muscles or joints?

Do you feel bad all over without any apparent cause?

Dr. Crook is a leading advocate of the candida yeast theory of medical illness. He asserts that if you answer five or six questions yes, your symptoms are probably yeast-connected. If you have three or four yes answers, then yeast possibly plays a role.

The candida theory of fatigue is to the 1980s what the hypoglycemia

* Adapted with permission from William Crook, *The Yeast Connection*, 3d ed. Jackson, Tenn.: Professional Books; New York: Vintage Books, 1986.

theory was to the 1950s: a medical breakthrough according to its believers; unscientific hogwash to the wary medical establishment.

I believe the candida theory has some applications to fatigue and other health problems. However, many candida advocates have oversold the theory, earning the justifiable ire of physicians and scientists. For example, consider this magazine ad for an "anti-Candida product":

". . . leading immunologists estimate that 80 million Americans . . . are already suffering from Candida Albicans."

It may sell medicines to the public, but it is not scientifically responsible.

The candida yeast theory stems from the work of Dr. C. Orian Truss, a Birmingham, Alabama, allergist. Dr. Truss noted that many patients with unexplained symptoms improved after treatments designed to control the candida yeast organism that normally shares our intestines. He believes candida yeast in the intestines may produce toxic elements that, when absorbed, can disturb the body's metabolism.

Since yeast flourishes in a high-sugar environment, Dr. Truss' treatment plan includes a low-sugar, low-carbohydrate diet much like the antihypoglycemia diet. In addition, Truss limits foods high in yeast such as bread, alcohol, vinegar products, dried fruit, aged cheeses, brewer's yeast, and mushrooms. He also prescribes a medicine, Nystatin, which (taken by mouth) destroys yeast in the intestine. Truss recommends that whenever feasible patients should avoid yeast-promoting medicines such as antibiotics, birth control pills, and adrenal steroid hormones (prednisone, cortisone).

Dr. Truss prescribes the anticandida treatment for several months. If improvement follows, he continues treatment for another three to nine months or even longer.

Since the publication of Dr. Truss' book *The Missing Diagnosis* and Dr. Crook's *The Yeast Connection,* the candida theory has received wide acceptance by nutrition commentators in the mass media, health food stores, and nonmainstream physicians. In contrast, the leading organizations of allergy physicians have condemned the theory as speculative and unproved.

Does the Candida Treatment Work?

Despite eloquent testimonials by doctors and patients, the candida advocates have not tested their treatment scientifically with untreated or placebo-treated patients to control for the effects of high hopes and enthusiasm.

Such studies would not be that difficult. Volunteers taking the standard candida treatment could be given a food supplement. Some would receive sugar, the others a non-yeast-promoting artificial sweetener. Both would be disguised so neither the patient nor the physician knew who had which. If the candida theory is correct, the volunteers receiving artificial sweetener should improve more rapidly than those receiving sugar. Other volunteers might receive an inert medicine instead of their Nystatin, or a candida-promoting medicine such as an antibiotic.

Because the candida advocates have not done this "homework," most physicians discount the treatment. My experience is more optimistic.

Several persons told me that Truss' treatment had helped them. I met Dr. Truss, Dr. Crook, and other leading candida supporters such as Dr. Sidney Baker of New Haven's Gesell Institute. I was impressed by their sincerity and intelligence and by the relative safety of their treatment plan.

I decided to offer Truss' program to selected patients after carefully explaining my skepticism. Most of the original patients improved. Four years later, my experience is that about 50 percent of patients who score high on Dr. Crook's quiz and who adopt the candida treatment program improve substantially. This might be due to a placebo effect, but it is a better result than I would expect from a placebo.

I believe it is legitimate to try the candida treatment, even though its effectiveness has not been proved. If properly supervised, the candida program should be extremely safe. A low-sugar, low-yeast diet is boring but nutritionally adequate. Nystatin, used at manufacturer's recommended doses, is less likely to cause serious harm than almost any other drug, including aspirin, Valium, and penicillin. In theory, prolonged use could cause one's yeast to develop resistance to Nystatin. However, so far as I can determine, no instances of this complication have yet been found.

To obtain a list of physicians in your area who use Dr. Truss' methods, contact either The Price-Pottenger Foundation, 5871 El Cajon Blvd., San Diego, CA 92115, or the International Health Foundation, Inc., P.O. Box 1000HF, Jackson, TN 38302. Both request a stamped self-addressed envelope and a $5 donation. Also discuss the candida program with your personal physician to ensure that the program's recommendations would be safe for you.

For best results, *work on your life stresses at the same time you pursue*

Suspect that the candida syndrome might contribute to your fatigue if:

- As a woman, you have a frequently recurring vaginal discharge that your doctor says is from candida yeast.
- You have had substantial exposure to such medicines that promote yeast as antibiotics, birth control pills, or adrenal steroid hormones.
- Your symptoms worsen with high intake of simple carbohydrate foods, (sugars, bread) or with foods containing yeast (vinegar, dried fruit, soy sauce, moldy cheese, such as Brie or Camembert) or improve on an antihypoglycemia or an anticandida diet.
- You have chronic irritable bowel syndrome: gas, diarrhea, constipation.
- You have various other complaints for which competent medical and psychiatric evaluation has determined no cause.

the candida program. Any chronic illness causes emotional suffering. However, many candida advocates also believe that emotional stress might increase one's vulnerability to the candida syndrome. One study showed that a high proportion of candida patients had traumatic childhood experiences such as loss of a parent, beating, or sexual abuse. I encourage "candida patients" to join our basic stress management program. If psychotherapy seems desirable, I refer to psychologists who respect patients' efforts to help themselves through the candida program.

Several Don'ts on Candida

Don't continue the candida treatment if it is clearly not working. A three-month trial of the diet and Nystatin should be enough to decide if there is a trend toward improvement. If not, seek another reason for your fatigue.

Don't rely entirely on doctors who make only "unorthodox" diagnoses, such as candida, vitamin deficiency, and hypoglycemia. If the only tool you have is a hammer, everything tends to look like a nail. Keep up with your regular physician for a periodic review.

Don't become a victim of the "candida terrors." Don't be terrified of eating even tiny portions of sugar or mold. Compulsive over-restriction is neither healthful nor necessary to achieve treatment goals to overcome candida.

Don't be misled by laboratory tests which claim to diagnose you as definitely having candida. Currently, there is no laboratory test that adequately predicts who will or will not respond to Truss' candida treatment. We all have candida in our bowel, skin, and often, microscopically, in our throats. Almost everyone reacts to candida on an allergy skin test. Blood tests can measure your level of antibody against candida, but we are not yet sure of their significance.

All candida medicines are not as safe as Nystatin. For example, Nizeral (ketoconazole) is a powerful antiyeast medicine that has a potential for damaging side effects. Its use requires liver-function and other blood tests to be monitored as frequently as every two or three weeks.

PART 2

MIND/BODY FACTORS THAT CAUSE FATIGUE

CHAPTER

6

STRESS

Carol H is a middle-level executive. She works very hard but gets little recognition. When the workday is over she has no energy left for her personal life.

Sandy D is the mother of twin eight-year-old girls. A perfectionist, she is vice-president of the PTA and sells real estate part-time. Her vigor is flagging and she doesn't know why.

John T is a respected and prosperous psychiatrist. At forty-five he doubts the value of his achievements and fights a daily battle against fatigue.

Jerry M was fired as vice-president of a computer company. Now, a year later, his finances are shaky but he feels very well as he struggles to build a business as a free-lance consultant.

These individuals are all under stress. Carol, Sandy, and John are worn out because of it. Jerry is not. This chapter examines why stress only sometimes causes fatigue—and when to suspect it is the cause of your symptoms.

Stress refers to demands or activities that stretch our ability to respond comfortably and describes the feeling of distress or negative tension that occurs because of such demands. These feelings can include anxiety, anger, boredom, or depression as well as the physical feelings of headache, irritable bowel, and chronic fatigue.

How Can You Tell If Your Fatigue Comes From Stress?

Insight into how stress causes fatigue can be gained by appreciating how your body responds to stressful situations. We have built into us a marvelous bodily system for survival, called the "fight/flight" response. Whenever we are in a perilous or arousing situation the body pours out adrenalin to brace us for action. It also triggers a variety of hormones and nerve impulse discharges that have dramatic effects. The heart pumps blood with extra speed and force so that muscles will be fully fueled and ready. The nervous system is activated so we are at high alert, can concentrate intently, and make rapid decisions. Blood-clotting factors are released so wounds won't bleed much. The entire organism is tense and poised to act.

When we had a simpler way of life we would strike at or run away from a snake, paddle our raft out of a fierce eddy, or deal with whatever emergency was presented. The event would end and the body would return to a normal, more relaxed state.

In the modern world life is often a series of stresses that arouse our bodies in the same fashion as a fight/flight emergency. You miss a bus, get stuck in traffic, the boss gives you a deadline of yesterday, household repair people don't show up, bills are higher than anticipated. Each of these stresses lasts a long time, without the relief of rapid resolution. And if you dislike your job, live in an unfriendly neighborhood, or have perpetual marital, children, or money problems, your stress may almost *never* abate. Your body is working full-time at a magnified intensity. *No wonder you are tired!*

Stress-response hormones produce emotional reactions, primarily anxiety. Stressful situations may also provoke anger, impatience, frustration, or depression and despair. These emotions can be clues that your body is bearing an overload, that it is time to take stock of your situation and improve it if you can. However, many individuals don't feel these emotions or don't recognize their meaning. They may be so accustomed to being worried or hostile that they think the condition is normal. But their nerves and hormones are reacting nevertheless, wearing them down physically and emotionally. Taxed to the limit, fatigue is inevitable—often with little awareness that stress is the villain.

An example of a person so used to his stress that he fails to perceive it is Hal Grey, a warm, generous fifty-five-year old who works as the chief custodian of a religious school. Four years ago his mother-in-law moved in with Hal and his wife. She was healthy, but "mainly sat in the house staring into space, not interested in anything."

Hal consulted me last year because of chronic fatigue. He improved 60 percent on a program of diet and exercise, but still did not feel like himself. Then a strange change occurred. His mother-in-law was stricken with cancer and became painfully bedridden. The demands of her terminal care were immense on both Hal and his wife. Yet as Hal struggled to comfort her, he recovered his energy.

"All those years I never realized how much I resented my mother-in-law's negative attitude and its effect on my home. But I couldn't express it even to myself. When she became sick, I felt sorry for her and I could see how angry I had been before." The stress of his mother-in-law's presence was the main reason for Hal's chronic fatigue. The greater stress of her terminal care was less fatiguing because it did not increase Hal's internal conflict—it actually healed it.

The tragic aspect of continuing stress is that it may be responsible for a multitude of ills. Headache, back pain, stomach disorders—even the common cold and serious infections such as tuberculosis are more likely to hit when the body is rendered vulnerable by stress. Stress reactions may foster heart disease by raising blood pressure, increasing cholesterol levels, causing narrowing or spasms of the main arteries of the heart, promoting undesirable blood clotting (thrombosis or embolism), upsetting the heart's rhythm and directly damaging the muscle of the heart. Stress' effect on the immune system may inhibit our defense against cancer as well.

Thus it is important to recognize stress overload and learn how to deal with it so you will not be constantly tired and will not become sick. Before discovering why Jerry M could escape stress despite his great troubles and how you can do the same, let's see how to tell if stress is why you are tired—physically, emotionally, or intellectually.

The first step is to recognize your sources of stress.

Make a wish list.

One way to identify stress is to write out a "wish list" of what your ideal life would be so you can compare it with your reality. For example, complete one of these sentences:

"My life would be perfect if—",

"If I could live my life over again, I would change—",

"I woke up today and all my problems were gone. This is what changed—".

Don't write what is practical or possible. Give yourself free rein. This list was written by John Talbot, a forty-six-year-old accountant, suburbanite, commuter, and father of three:

> There would be a 26-hour day so I could get more sleep and time to myself.
>
> I'd use a Star-Trek transporter so I could be at work in seconds instead of an hour.
>
> I'd no longer wait at the Lincoln Tunnel.

I'd have time to exercise every day. I'd never feel rushed.

My wife wouldn't criticize me when I come home late, when I want to go bowling, when I don't wear the clothes she likes. She would treat me like a prince, the way she did before the kids were born.

My boss would get off my back. I'd be the boss. . . . No, I don't want that. . . . I'll win the lottery. What would I do then? Retire? Coach baseball? Sounds like fun. If I had a million dollars, would life be easier? Sure it would. Maybe I'd work part time.

How will I put three kids through college? I can't afford that.

Is my son Tommy getting into drugs? I wish he were happier.

I wish my wife wouldn't always be too tired for sex. I guess I haven't been showing her much warmth either.

I smoke too much. It isn't good for me. I'm getting old. I wish I were thirty again, and knew all I know now. What's the point? Do I just keep commuting for the next twenty years?

John felt pressured by his responsibilities. Career satisfaction, which had sustained him before, was no longer enough. Personal and family life were underdeveloped.

As John read his list, he saw the pattern that was draining his energy.

As his understanding increased, John considered his options. He thought about changing jobs to be nearer home, but decided he needed the higher pay in the city until the children were through college. He began exercising during lunch hour. He felt pleased to see himself getting into shape. He discussed his frustration with his wife, and learned of her wishes and needs that had not been met. They are making genuine efforts to improve their relationship and are beginning to draw close again.

Six months later, John has a better sense of who he is and what he wants. While life is not perfect, he has more energy now that he is confronting his stresses with purpose, even those stresses he is not in a position to change.

THE QUANTITY OF STRESS

A second way to identify stress is to take inventory of life situations that are frequently its sources. Stress comes in big packages and little ones.

Major changes in life circumstances increase vulnerability to stress-induced physical and emotional disorders, including fatigue. Major life changes have been linked to an increased risk of heart attack, diabetes, stomach ulcers, chronic yeast infections, tuberculosis, depression, and decreased performance in jobs and at school. Recent research indicates that people suffering death of a spouse develop measurable reductions in key cells of their immune system.

The surprise is that even positive changes can be stressful: having a baby, an outstanding achievement, buying a new house, gaining a promotion at work, taking a vacation. Changes that are most strongly predictive of subsequent difficulty include death of a close family member, divorce or marital separation, getting married, being fired, retirement, a serious injury or illness, or difficulty with the law. Just below these in impact are pregnancy and childbirth, marital reconciliation, illness of a family member, sexual difficulties, changing jobs, a child leaving home, taking a large mortgage. Other life changes that cause stress include any change in living circumstances, beginning or ending school, trouble with the boss, trouble with in-laws, change in the number of arguments with spouse, change in responsibilities at work, change in social, family, or recreational activities.

If your life has changed for good or for ill during the six months before you became fatigued consider stress as a possible cause. Of course certain life changes happen to all of us; some are highly predictable. These normal transitions (such as that from young adulthood into middle age) are times of special psychological vulnerability when unexpected changes and routine life stresses can have extraordinary impact—causing chronic fatigue as one of many potential problems. These stages of growth and maturing are discussed in Chapter 7.

However, most stress is not from major life changes. It consists of "small stuff" that goes on every day—particularly the small stuff we are unable to change. A sense of lacking control over circumstances is a major source of stress. One startling example is the fact that policemen rate as most stressful "distorted or negative press accounts of police" and "ineffectiveness of the judicial system." Reading the newspaper or sitting safely in court was perceived as more stressful than responding to a felony in progress or making an arrest while alone. The last are events they can influence; news accounts and courts are beyond their control.

Researchers have shown the critical importance of a sense of control by studying its effects on experimental animals. In one classic study two rats are given stressful electric shocks. One has the opportunity to prevent the shocks to both when he succeeds in moderately difficult challenges such as jumping over a bar. When he fails, both are punished. Although both receive identical shocks, the first rat partly controls his own fate. The second rat cannot. Usually the first rat remains healthy and energetic. The passive rat becomes listless and ill, with stomach ulcer and death being common results. The brain of the passive rat shows a decrease in chemical transmitters in the pattern expected for depression. Transmitter levels in the active rat remain high.

Office workers' complaints reflect a need for a sense of control; their most stressful complaints include inadequate support from supervisors, excessive paperwork, lack of recognition for good work, lack of participation in policy decisions, too much work pressure, too little salary, problems with co-workers, and trouble with supervisors. There are few stresses worse than constantly feeling "dumped on."

Studies of civil service workers in England find greater feelings of stress and higher rates of heart disease among low-level workers than among administrators, even when smoking, diet, and other heart risks were the same; lack of control over job tasks may be the critical factor. Other studies confirm that workers who put up with many demands and control few decisions suffer most from stress-induced disorders. Work you hate can make you tired.

Having *too little* stress is another stress-related problem. Many persons lack worthy, interesting, or important challenges. Such understimulation is also a stress. With too little challenge, life can lose its sense of purpose.

YOUR EMOTIONAL REACTION TO STRESS

Stress itself is only part of the problem. More important is how you react to it. Some people have punishing emotional reactions that seem to feed on themselves, becoming an additional source of chronic distress. Other people are like the proverbial ducks—water rolls off their backs instead of drenching them. Events don't upset their emotional equilibrium. Table 6.1 lists feelings that people who have a problem with stress often experience. Read through them quickly, checking which ones often affect you. If these negative emotions tend to dominate your life, look carefully for your sources of stress. They are probably contributing to your fatigue.

Anger, anxiety, and depression are the most common and important stress-related emotions.

Anger may be the most lethal emotion. Type A (hurried, hard-driving, competitive) personalities have heart attacks at a very high rate.

Recent research indicates that the angry, impatient hostility that lies at the core of many Type As may be the main reason. Such anger or hostility can also keep you fatigued.

Do you become furious when you are slowed by traffic? Do you often fly off the handle? Do you nurture a grievance or hold on to a grudge? Are you impatient with others' mistakes or shortcomings?

An intense anger response is a habit you can change. But first you must recognize its role.

Anxiety is the most common stress reaction. Produced by adrenalin-type stimulant hormones, anxiety winds you up and wears you down. It is often the cause of chronic fatigue.

Anxiety—basically a free-floating fear—causes nervousness, worried anticipation, explosive angry reactions, and other disturbing behaviors. It can also resemble a physical disease. Anxious people almost always suffer symptoms from at least three of the following four categories:

1. *Symptoms resulting from physical muscle tension or activity*—jitteriness, trembling, set jaw with gritted teeth, muscle heaviness or ache, easy tiring, eyelid-twitching, furrowed brow, fidgeting, restlessness.

2. *Symptoms caused by overactivation of the nervous system*—heart pounding, cold or clammy hands, dry mouth, dizziness or light-headedness, numbness or tingling hands or feet, upset stomach, hot or cold spells, frequent urination, diarrhea, stomach discomfort, lump in throat, flushing, paleness, rapid pulse or breathing.

3. *Apprehension or fearful expectations*—feeling anxious or worried about the future, anticipating that something bad is imminent (that you might faint, lose control, have an accident). Such fears can be intense and frequent.

4. *Symptoms caused by hyperalertness*—scanning for danger, poor concentration, impatience, difficulty sleeping.

Of course, everyone experiences some of these occasionally, but if you experience them a lot the strain of anxiety probably contributes to your fatigue.

There are periods in life when some anxiety is predictable. This adjustment anxiety results from life's normal stresses: the teenager's transition into adulthood, career changes, moving, retirement, physical illness, and so on. Adjustment anxiety responds particularly well to counseling, so recognizing it is especially important.

General anxiety is the most common form of anxiety, but special

Table 6.1: NEGATIVE FEELINGS THAT CAN BE A CLUE TO STRESS

Anger	Worry	Self-centeredness
Hostility	Anxiety	Selfishness
Suspicion	Fear of losing control	Uncaring
Impatience	Fright	Guilt
Overcompetitiveness	Loneliness	Worthlessness
Disorganization	Unfulfillment	Sensitivity
Impulsivity	Boredom	Rejection
Unsureness	Sadness	Helplessness
Unassertiveness	Staleness	Exploitedness
Indecisiveness	Spiritlessness	Lack of appreciation
Rigidity	Emptiness	Humiliation
Overstrictness	Undersexed	Bitterness
Perfectionism	Oversexed	Unloved

kinds can also result in fatigue. Panic anxiety triggers sudden fear, terror, or a sense of impending doom, often with physical symptoms such as shortness of breath, hyperventilation, palpitations, shakiness, or confusion. Obsessive-compulsive anxiety features irresistible ideas, thoughts, or impulses or stereotyped motions such as hand-washing, counting, checking, or touching. Phobic anxiety triggers fear in open places, crowds, tunnels, and social or other situations. Post-traumatic stress anxiety repeats in thought, dream, or bodily symptoms traumatic events from the recent or distant past such as war experiences, auto accidents, childhood beatings, sexual abuse, or the death of a loved one.

Anxiety can occur for physical reasons as well: too little sleep, overactive thyroid, heart arrhythmia, chronic lung disease, low potassium or magnesium, hidden infection. Of course, any illness that creates worry or pain can cause anxiety indirectly. Sometimes medicines are also anxiety stimulators (among them asthma medicines, nasal decongestants, and diet pills that contain caffeine), as are tobacco and alcohol as well as illegal stimulants such as cocaine and amphetamines.

Depression is the third key emotion triggered by stress. It is so important a cause of fatigue that it has a chapter of its own, Chapter 8.

IDENTIFY STRESS BY CURING IT

There is one excellent way to decide if stress is responsible for your tiredness: reduce it and see if you improve.

You don't need a year's psychotherapy. Often simpler steps can give you the answer. For example:

Take a vacation (or send your teenagers or in-laws on one). Feeling better on vacation and worse when you return is a good cue that the stress is too great at work, in your home, or in your daily routine. Of course other factors also change on vacation: diet, allergic exposure, sleep. Nevertheless, if you do improve on vacation suspect that less stress may be the reason.

Start a gentle but steady exercise program. Exercise often alleviates stress. Try it five days a week for a trial period of six weeks. If you feel better after you exercise—less stressed, less anxious, less depressed—or feel worse when you skip a day, stress may be part of your fatigue problem.

If you get worse with exercise, stress or anxiety can still be a factor. Some people with general anxiety and perhaps 30 percent of individuals with the panic-disorder form of anxiety worsen during exercise.

Take a course of relaxation or stress management. Visual imagery, yoga, meditation, pleasant music, or massage can tone down your body's reaction to stress. We run a four- to six-session stress management program as part of our medical practice. We can teach almost anyone how to relax. If someone learns to relax and relaxation fails to affect symptoms, we can be fairly confident that stress probably is not the problem.

For a quickie version of a relaxation technique, try this:

Close your eyes, withdrawing your attention into yourself.

Allow the muscles of your mouth and eyes to form a gentle smile.

Say to yourself "My mind and my body are relaxing."

Breathe slowly and deeply, free and easy, let the muscles of your abdomen move gently, in and out.

As you exhale, relax your jaw, your forehead, and the muscles of your neck and shoulders.

Feel a wave of warmth and gentleness pass down to your toes.

Repeat, as desired, enjoying this feeling of calm relaxation.

Open your eyes, feeling refreshed and alert, ready to resume your normal activities.

Appendix 4 contains several relaxation exercises and a selection of relaxation tapes.

Consider a trial of treatment using a tranquilizer. I rarely prescribe tranquilizers such as Valium and Librium for long-term treatment because they can be habit-forming. However, a two-week trial of antianxiety medicine makes sense as a diagnostic technique. If you feel better after that time, you probably suffer from anxiety. Unfortunately, most antianxiety medicines sedate while they relax—so if you are already tired antianxiety medicines might make you worse. BuSpar (buspirone), a new antianxiety medicine, is not habit-forming and is nonsedating.

Obtain a short course of psychological counseling. Traditional psychotherapy tends to be prolonged. In recent years, however, many psychologists have adopted techniques that yield improvement within ten or twelve sessions. A diagnostic trial of brief psychotherapy often makes sense.

Reducing Stress

If these approaches give good indication that stress is the cause of your tiredness, relaxation training is but one way to deal with it. There are actually four basic strategies: change the situations that stress you; adopt stress-resistant patterns of thinking and acting; understand yourself psychologically to reduce your stress vulnerability; and train your mind and body to be relaxed and resilient so that stresses and disappointments will not hit you so hard.

1. CHANGING YOUR SITUATION

Stress specialists know that it's not the stressor that gets a person down but rather how well he or she deals with it. The simplest stress-reduction technique is learning to say no. Overcommitment inevitably means stress, even if each single activity is desirable by itself. Anything ceases to be fun if it turns you into a pressure cooker. Identify your values and priorities, because saying no means you will have to pick and choose. If you are competitive and take on every challenge that comes along, you need to practice letting some pass.

Set aside time for yourself—for rest, enjoyment, thinking. Set aside time for a few important personal relationships. Many stress-prone people feel guilty and fidgety when not working or "doing something." Do things, but things you enjoy, that calm you down.

Organize your day and your future commitments as well. Schedule fewer appointments. Stop wearing your watch or tuning in to news reports that remind you of the time and feed your sense of time-pressure. With a less cluttered agenda and a clearer focus you will work more efficiently and recognize when you are beginning to overload. Are there more efficient or pleasant ways to accomplish a task? Can you car-pool the kids instead of driving yourself? Might a chore become fun if you do it with a friend? Should you spend more money to save time or more time to save money?

Can you disarm or forgive your interpersonal conflicts? Might Hal Gray have changed his mother-in-law's behavior had he discussed it with her initially? Perhaps he would have learned that his mother-in-law was depressed. Certainly it would have helped *him* to have expressed his negative feelings instead of bottling them inside.

2. STRESS-RESISTANT BEHAVIOR AND ATTITUDES

Stress researchers agree that the more you can count on emotional support from caring friends and family, the more resistant you will be to stress. Lack of a soft shoulder or willing ear increases stress vulnerability. It is astonishing to what extent pouring out your distressing predicament really does relieve the load. One study found that stress was appreciably reduced simply by having people devote a half-hour to writing down things they were ashamed of, that they'd never revealed to anyone. Just putting it "outside themselves" on paper lightened the burden.

People at high risk for feeling isolated include children who feel their parents won't listen; the corporate spouse who relocates to a strange town every two years; the chronically ill individual whose family and friends think its "all in your head"; the older person who becomes socially cut off. Persons who lack a network of people they can count on are more likely to lose their energy or become depressed, even at levels of stress that most would consider relatively mild. People who are not linked meaningfully to others have far higher death rates than those who are. Fatigue long precedes these tragic outcomes.

Our friend Jerry M, the computer consultant, bounced back from being fired in part because he had a fundamental belief in himself and in part because he was blessed with a very supportive wife. She remained cheerful and encouraging, helping Jerry overcome his initial feelings of humiliation. Jerry also had good friends who listened, encouraged, and shared accounts of their own business reversals. They also introduced Jerry to potential new clients.

Who can you count on to listen or help when you have a problem? Family is valuable, but spouse, parents, and children are often affected by the same stresses that you are. Siblings who live separately, other relatives, friends, and co-workers can really lend support.

It's never too late for you to broaden or deepen your friendships. Develop interests that involve you with people. Reach out to others, especially when they are in need. You will feel better for it, and it can pay you back handsomely when you need support. Good friends can help you withstand the stresses that cause fatigue.

Being involved and interested in hobbies or activities also provides armor against stress. For example, involvement with a pet increases feelings of satisfaction and well-being. This is especially true for people, such as shut-ins, who have limited social involvement. Even taking care of a houseplant has been shown to increase energy and interest among residents of nursing homes.

Negative habits of thinking lead to trouble. An entire school of psychology called cognitive therapy is devoted to recognizing and correcting unrealistically negative perceptions. Do you jump to conclusions too quickly? For example, "Jane hasn't called me in a week. She must be angry at me." Do you overgeneralize? "*Nothing* ever turns out right!" Do you take things too personally? "Everyone kept staring at me—I must look a mess." Do you ignore the good side and see only the bad? Do you get trapped into "either/or" thinking so that if you don't accomplish everything you want you feel like a total failure?

In contrast, adopting positive attitudes and habits of thinking promotes stress-resistance. When faced with trouble ask yourself "Is this trouble really worth all the fuss?" (As one leading stress researcher puts it: "Rule one is 'Don't sweat the small stuff.' Rule two—'It's (almost) all small stuff.' ") Am I expecting too much of others? Am I expecting too much of myself? Am I being too sensitive? Can I ignore small frustrations instead of letting them take control? Can I accept the advice of the English novelist G. K. Chesterton?: 'An adventure is an inconvenience rightly considered. An inconvenience is an adventure wrongly considered' "

Another way to avoid stress and have a more fulfilling life is to cultivate "hardiness." We talked about how workers suffer from having many job demands but little control over policy. The hardy personality doesn't passively accept everything thrown at him or her. This type of survivor attempts constructive input—not griping, which only feeds the bitter sense of enslavement, but positive influence on what he or she does. What's more, the hardy personality doesn't view each task as an imposition. Instead, responsibilities are accepted with some enthusiasm, as an interesting challenge. Hardy people basically enjoy their work. My advice: Select work you like or find something to like in the work you do, whether in factory, office, or home. There are rewards in every undertaking, from fixing a leak, to sealing ten thousand envelopes, to attempting to sell a customer on the merits of a product. You can take pride in the zeal you bring to any task.

Cultivate an optimistic sense that you are in control of your life. Is the glass half full or half empty? The glass doesn't decide. The choice is yours. If you are in the habit of looking down, practice looking up for a while. Some of the favorite self-hypnosis sentences of the patients in our stress management program sound corny but are remarkably effective: My self-confidence is increasing. I am in control. I deserve to be happy. My energy is increasing.

Success builds on itself. Set up small challenges at which you can succeed. In a fascinating study of biofeedback treatment for tension headaches, volunteers were given either true biofeedback (showing the actual tension in their forehead muscles) or false biofeedback (unrelated to their muscle tension). Half the people in each group were given enthusiastic encouragement, told how wonderfully they were doing, and assured that they would certainly succeed in reducing their headaches. The others were given only moderate praise.

The high-expectation patients did dramatically better than the low-expectation ones. Whether they received actual biofeedback or false information made no difference. Moral: Creating the expectation of improvement is most of the battle.

THE ROLE OF PSYCHOTHERAPY OR COUNSELING

If you suspect you have unresolved issues from developmental crises or if you feel affected by emotions you do not understand, you might feel better after a period of reflection or discussion with a particularly trustworthy friend. However, psychological counseling may be a more efficient approach, especially if similar problems or feelings have plagued you for years.

Your personal physician or an acquaintance who has been helped are your best initial sources for selecting a counselor or therapist. Psychiatrists, psychologists, social workers, and pastoral counselors can do psychotherapy. I prefer first an evaluation with a psychiatrist or a highly recommended Ph.D. psychologist, since they are particularly skilled in evaluating whether treatment is needed and which kind would be best. However, when it comes to ongoing therapy, which may last for months or for years, I find the therapist's degrees are much less important than the chemistry of your interpersonal relationship.

There are several schools of psychotherapy, and they differ in their approach. However, many studies have shown that even these differences are less important than the overriding issue of whether or not you feel involved in your relationship with the therapist. These issues are discussed further in Chapter 8.

TRAINING YOURSELF TO BE RELAXED AND RESILIENT

As the song writer Johnny Mercer said: "You've got to Ac-Cent-Tchu-Ate the positive, E-lim-my-nate the neg-a-tive, Latch on to the affirm-a-tive . . . ."

Many of us are in the habit of overreacting. Fortunately, several strategies can tone down the distress we cause by overreacting to stressful events. Relaxation exercises, guided visual imagery, meditation, yoga, biofeedback, spiritual centering, and self-hypnosis all train the mind and body to react calmly to life's challenges and demands.

I began stress management-relaxation training in my medical practice four years ago. I wish I had known about it from the beginning. It has worked wonders for many patients who suffer from stress and fatigue. Other stress management approaches include physical exercise, getting adequate sleep, proper nutrition, and spiritual involvement.

Most stress management techniques are easy to learn. Best results are obtained with a qualified trainer. Appendix 4 contains several useful relaxation exercises.

THE MAIN OBSTACLE TO STRESS MANAGEMENT: FEELING HOPELESS AND TRAPPED

The biggest obstacle to coping with stress is the belief that you cannot change your situation or your energy-robbing emotional reactions.

Beverly T was tired because of chronic stress. Married unhappily, she had no children and did not work. Her seventy-year-old mother lived with her.

Beverly's fatigue was worse when she ate high-sugar foods or drank alcohol. She improved 25 percent with an antihypoglycemia diet. A medical examination showed her to be physically normal. The rest of her problem seemed due to stress.

Beverly had wanted children, but her husband had been unwilling. At thirty-eight she considered herself too old and deeply resented her husband for imposing this decision on her. She no longer cared for him but was unwilling to divorce because she felt financially dependent. Beverly's mother was in good health but became upset whenever Beverly left the house. Beverly spent most of her time watching television with her mother.

Beverly was trapped. She resented both her dependence on her husband and her mother's demands, but she could not choose an alternative. She could barely acknowledge her anger and frustration, much less express it. This was a tremendous drain on her energy.

Beverly had several options, none perfect. She could upgrade her job skills to seek financial independence. However, she doubted that even upgraded skills could command the salary she needed for the life-style she wanted. She could enter marital counseling to rebuild her relationship with her husband. She rejected this because she bore too strong a grudge to let go of her anger. She could seek a deeper reason for her anger through psychotherapy, but Beverly felt that since her anger was justified psychotherapy could be of no value. Beverly understood the price she was paying to maintain her status quo, but she seemed to prefer her distress to any alternative.

For the first three months after our conversation, she consulted several "vitamin specialists" seeking a biological quick fix to reverse her fatigue. However, despite her initial rejection of the possibility of change, she also took steps to escape from her trap.

Despite her mother's objections Beverly took a part-time job as a sales clerk. She enjoyed the social interaction on the job and the excuse it gave to be out of the house. She did well at the job and her self-confidence increased. She is now taking a night course in bookkeeping to upgrade her work skills. She also renewed a childhood interest in drama, participating in small roles with a local theatre group. She has not moved closer to her husband, but as she adds new interests, her anger and frustration seem less important. At the same time, she has been less bothered by fatigue.

Beverly's story shows that even unchangeable situations can usually be changed—not to perfection, but for the better.

CHAPTER

7

LIFE CYCLE VULNERABILITY CRISES

Just as critical life events such as marriage and losing or starting a job can be severely taxing, there are also transition periods in everyone's life that increase our vulnerability to stress-induced fatigue. These are the turning points between developmental periods—childhood, adolescence, young adulthood, middle age, and old age.

During the periods of transition, the individual is pulled in opposing directions, like a quivering metal object between two magnets: the safe dependency of childhood versus the adolescent drive to be free of control; a secure job versus unfulfilled aspirations; career obligations versus home and family; personal obligations versus personal fulfillment.

These yearnings, tugging in different directions, may have a net effect of exhaustion. Fatigue may mean physically, emotionally, as well as symbolically "I am not yet ready, willing, or able to make this difficult choice." A feeling of collapse extricates you from the fray.

Much unexplained fatigue is the unhappy result of "normal" external stress at a time of special emotional vulnerability. Understanding where you are in your psychological passage can provide valuable clues to why you are suffering.

THE ADOLESCENT CRISIS: AGE SIXTEEN TO TWENTY-TWO

As teenagers we tread the unsteady path from childhood dependence on home, parents, and friends toward an adult sense of independence and purpose. At points during this period the pot comes to boil as the adolescent tries on and sheds various answers to the questions "Who am I?" "What do I want?" Popularly known as the identity crisis, this can be an extremely vulnerable period psychologically.

Jean was a college drop-out at twenty. The youngest child of a loving middle-class family, Jean became disoriented while trying to "find" herself. After a period with drugs and promiscuous sex during which ill health was a constant companion, she is now seeking a more constructive direction. A newly passionate environmentalist, she plans to return to college hoping for a career in environmental law.

At core, Jean is a normal kid who has passed through rough times. With reasonable luck, she will find her course, only a few years behind schedule. Adolescent crises need not be so dramatic, but a turbulent period of self-questioning often makes for a healthy transition to the next stage of life.

Fatigue may set in when the identity crisis is long or intense. Failure to complete the identity crisis, or failure to attempt it, is a prescription for prolonged immaturity and distressing self-doubt that may carry forward, even for decades. Chronic fatigue is only one of its symptoms. If you are older but still feel adolescent, psychological counseling might be extremely valuable in helping you move on.

YOUNG ADULTHOOD: LOOKING FOR MEANING IN WORK AND IN LOVE

In their twenties, most people establish tentative adult commitments—to a career, to another individual, to a system of values. These roles are in part what we want for ourselves but are still heavily influenced by what we feel parents, peer groups, and the general culture expect.

If you are in your twenties, where do you stand with commitment? Did you commit before you were sure? Regret over paths unexplored can produce dissatisfaction and fatigue as one labors without desire—or with conflicting goals. Have you been unwilling to commit, drifting from job to job or relationship to relationship without sinking roots? This path promotes uncertainty or isolation that undermines one's sense of purpose and energy.

John K is twenty-eight, but has not made a commitment. He worked in Africa for the Peace Corps from ages twenty-one to twenty-three, returning for graduate studies in political science. Dropping out after one year, he has held a dozen jobs, none of which seemed interesting or important enough to pursue for long. Good-looking and gregarious, John never lacked for girlfriends, but he has never established a mature, caring, intimate relationship. He feels empty inside, isolated from his friends who established roots, and disappointed that he has not yet "grown up." A lack of commitment is at the core of John's long-standing fatigue. John would also benefit from psychotherapy, to help him define his goals as well as reasonable paths to achieving them. His fatigue and "lack of drive" are less the cause of his problems than they are the natural effects of deep-seated indecision.

AGE THIRTY: THE MINI-MIDLIFE CRISIS

If you are about thirty, you have probably focused so long on getting started or getting ahead that you may wonder if important aspects of life might be passing you by. If you have been dedicated to career, you may long for marriage and family. If you are a housewife/mother, you may crave contact with the "real" world. The work or the marriage that was once exciting and fulfilling may by age thirty seem dull or routine.

The Mancinis are in marriage counseling. Tom at thirty-two is "making it" in a Wall Street law firm. He is at the office fifty hours a week and always brings work home. Barbara, twenty-nine, worked as a secretary to support Tom through law school, then "retired" to the suburbs to raise children and care for a home, she thought, for the rest of her life. To Tom, Barbara has lost the zest and interest she had when they married. Barbara feels trapped in the "mind-numbing world of house, children, and carpool." Their sex life is vacant. Neither has energy by the end of the day.

The task of age thirty is to review one's commitments to be sure they still serve your needs as your perspective lengthens, and your values mature. Age thirty often involves risk-taking such as career change and /or divorce. Or it can lead to a more meaningful commitment to the same job or spouse. Either way, facing the "crisis" is an energy drain. Ignoring the crisis only makes matters worse, since such issues, unconfronted, remain a chronic source of psychological stress.

TIME RUNNING OUT: THE MIDLIFE MALAISE

Somewhere between the late thirties or early forties most of us begin to sense that we are mortal. We realize we might not attain the goals of our twenties and thirties, and we become less sure of the importance of these goals. We recognize that we have neglected key aspects of life as we pursued others. Our time left is limited, yet we are still incomplete. Is this all there is? Can we be more?

Terry D was in a rut. At forty-four he was one of three vice-presidents of a large company. Yet the career ambition, which had been the center of his life, seemed stale. He was tired all the time. He had no zest for business. Two years ago he made a desperate effort to make life more interesting and himself more alive psychologically. A turn for the erratic: alcohol first, then an extramarital affair, finally a fling at mountain climbing that nearly ended in disaster. He suddenly understood. He had tried to turn back the clock because he did not feel good about the course of his life.

Terry liked his job, but that wasn't enough. Where were his idealistic dreams to make the world a better place? When had he lost the tender feelings he once had for his wife? How could he replace those weekends he had not spent with his children, who were now nearly grown? He felt his successes were hollow, that in a sense he had failed. He was tired, anxious, and a little depressed.

Terry worked through his crisis. He stayed at his job, but with better perspective. Some colleagues claimed he had lost his toughness; others said he was less a machine and more of a person. He spent evenings and weekends with his wife and his children. He took on the chairmanship of the social action committee at church. Weekend bicycle trips replaced mountain climbing.

Terry's sense of well-being returned and with it his confidence and stamina. Becoming president of his company seemed less likely, but this was more than balanced by his renewed sense of purpose in life.

If you are at midlife you need to take stock of where you have been and where you are going. If you don't do it consciously, your unconscious will. For those with careers like Terry, you may find a need to develop your caring and creative sides. For housewives and mothers who have been caring for others, it may be time for more selfishness to fulfill neglected personal needs for intellectual or economic productivity.

Although often unsettling, the reward of reassessing your direction at midlife is renewed strength of purpose and energy for life. Ignoring this crisis and its need to rebalance often leads to a sense of stagnation, which can be perceived as indistinguishable from fatigue.

THE POST-MIDDLE YEARS AND THE CRISIS OF AGING

As the saying goes, growing old is pretty bad, except when you consider the alternative. However, contrary to what you might think, despite illness and the loss of parents or friends, many people find their post-midlife-crisis years, say forty-five to seventy and beyond, among the best years of their lives. Whether one feels energetic and enthusiastic or tired and withdrawn depends in part on how well the person has come to terms with his or her reality. Often one feels more secure in who he or she is, acts more on individual initiative and less to make an impression. Men deepen their friendships and develop the "feminine" virtues of sharing and expressing emotions. Women become more assertive and worldly. Many of us develop a clearer sense of what really matters. Such people can have remarkable get-up-and-go. Others, who feel beaten by life, can become listless TV watchers or immobile sufferers of fatigue.

As old age approaches with the eventual certainty of death, we face another psychological crisis. Do we continue to live life to the full or feel as if life has already ended? Do we maintain an interest in the future, for our children, friends, country, and world? Or do we lapse into cynicism, isolation, or despair? At its best old age leads to a sense of personal integrity and wisdom; the alternative leads to a sense of helplessness, dogmatic opinionism, or disdain. The former invigorates; the latter fatigues. Which path you take depends in part on events over which we have only partial control: health, finances, family relationships. However, much depends also on where we are psychologically. Therefore, improving self-knowledge through self-reflection or through counseling can make a difference in how well we live.

Isaac D was a socialist in his youth but a career civil servant as an adult. The longer he lived the fewer his illusions. Now, in his late seventies, his strong opinions are ossified and his skepticism has degenerated into cynicism. His main joy is argument and criticizing the weaknesses of mankind. His children visit out of obligation. His wife puts up with him out of necessity. As Isaac became increasingly irascible, he grew more isolated and discouraged. What might have been his golden years of educating grandchildren, advocating social improvement, or refining his philosophical views did not materialize. While to outsiders a perverse and argumentative vigor remained, what Isaac experienced primarily was weariness: world-weariness and self-contempt for his ineffectual position.

FINDING YOURSELF IN YOUR LIFE CYCLE

Your age tells you approximately which developmental "crises" you have been through as well as which you are in or about to enter. Don't assume you are the exception. One way or other the critical issues of life's great transitions confront everyone.

Appendix 5 provides a panoramic overview of these issues. Your answers to this questionnaire may stimulate your reflection on where you have been and where you want to go.

If you suspect that unresolved issues continue to stress you, or if you feel caught in emotions you do not understand, you will probably feel better after a period of serious self-reflection or of sharing discussions with a very trustworthy friend. However, psychological counseling is often a more efficient approach, especially if similar problems or feelings have plagued you for years.

CHAPTER

8

DEPRESSION

Sarah was depressed and knew it. She was tired, so tired that she did not care to get up even after a night's sleep. She had children and a husband who loved her, but she blamed herself for not achieving her life's goals. All she used to enjoy—children, hobbies, exercise, sex—had lost their attractiveness. She felt hopeless and cried without reason. She wondered whether life was worth the effort to go on.

Fortunately, Sarah's husband realized she was suffering from depression. Sarah agreed, and although she was not optimistic, accepted a consultation with a psychiatrist. Sarah's tiredness was easily recognizable as the result of her depressed mood.

Helen was depressed but did *not* know it. She too was tired, but Helen didn't feel sad. Instead, her sleep was restless; she woke early and could not return to sleep. Food held no interest. Every day something else went wrong—headaches, backaches, nausea, constipation, cramps. As her health deteriorated she lost touch with her friends. Her household tasks seemed never to get done. She wondered if she were becoming senile. Of course she felt depressed at times; but with her health problems, she thought, who wouldn't?

Helen saw a gastroenterologist for her constipation, an orthopedist for her back, and a neurologist about her headaches. Could it be thyroid, she wondered? Should she take vitamins?

Her family physician pointed out that physical symptoms such as fatigue, lack of energy, stomach distress, headaches, and muscle soreness, particularly together, are common among people who suffer from depression.

This didn't make sense to Helen. She wasn't imagining her pains and lack of energy. Her husband was incensed. To him a "mental" illness was an embarrassment. Was the doctor saying that Helen is crazy?

Over the next visits, Helen was reassured that depression is not "all in your head." Depression is a disease that affects the body as much as the mind.

Helen and Sarah both recovered their energy within a few months of proper treatment. But Helen suffered six months longer before her depression was recognized. An estimated nine million people in the United States suffer depression; most are not diagnosed and treated. Almost all are dispirited or tired. The main goal of this chapter is to enable you to recognize when your fatigue is the result of depression. You will also learn how to avoid being diagnosed as depressed if this is not the case. Physicians, family, and friends sometimes assume depression must be the problem when no other reason for tiredness is found.

The essential features of depression are a mood of ill-feeling or dissatisfaction together with loss of interest or pleasure in usual activities. In the classic case one feels sad, blue, hopeless, low, discouraged, worthless, guilt-ridden, or down in the dumps. Such people, like Sarah, are usually recognized promptly and referred to a specialist.

But many with depression feel only a vague dissatisfaction or loss of energy, perhaps with a variety of physical complaints. Like Helen, they are more likely to visit their family physician than see a psychiatrist. They most often complain of fatigue; decreased *or* increased appetite; weight loss or weight gain; difficulty sleeping *or* excessive sleeping; anxiety and increased body activity *or* decreased body movement and speech; loss of ability to think clearly, concentrate, or make decisions.

Bodily symptoms may include headaches; muscle and joint aches; dizziness; nausea; constipation; abdominal cramps and intestinal gas. These "symptoms of depression" also occur with many other illnesses, as well as among healthy individuals—which is why depression is so easily overlooked or misunderstood.

Recognizing depression is not an exact science. Blood tests to diagnose it are not perfected, and no brain-wave machine can measure it accurately. The diagnosis is confirmed over time if improvement follows proper treatment.

If, like Helen, you feel tired and have a list of bodily complaints for which no cause can be found, ask yourself "Might depression be the cause?" If your enthusiasm for life has also waned, definitely consider depression as a cause. As a practical matter, *all* people who are chronically tired should ask themselves seriously whether depression might be part of their problem.

When Should You Suspect You May Be Depressed?

There are three main components to the illness of depression: (1) a sad, disappointed, or depressed mood; (2) loss of interest or pleasure in usual activities; (3) associated symptoms such as fatigue.

If your mood is depressed—sad, hopeless, worthless, or just "don't care," you have depression and your depression is a likely contributor to your fatigue. This is true *even* if a separate illness is the cause of the depression. People suffering strokes often become depressed. Although this is an understandable response to a serious illness, depressed stroke victims do better if the depression is specifically recognized and treated.

If you are not in touch with feelings of depression but no longer look forward to doing what you used to do, depression could be the reason. Many people who lose touch with their friends or family blame it on lack of energy or not feeling well. Often this is really a disguised way of saying that one no longer enjoys the people or things one did before. If you find yourself doing less and seeing fewer people, this could be a clue to an underlying depression.

Depressed people may feel they cannot afford to buy things, even though they have ample funds. They may be pessimistic—convinced that whatever they try will not work out. They often blame themselves for things that are not within their control. They are sometimes chronically angry, but usually most angry at themselves. Sex and love may seem to disappear. Or they may become "oversexed" to enjoy brief highs or to feel alive and loved. Most often, they are just weary. Nothing seems worth the effort.

Of course, some people limit their activity but are not depressed. For example, Susan is a woman with a recurring low-grade virus infection known as the chronic Epstein-Barr virus syndrome. Some days she is so wiped out she can hardly do anything. This gets her down. But depression is not her primary illness because Susan hates it when her activity is limited. She loves to be active, and on days when she feels physically well she is out doing everything. Even when she is physically down she tries to do the things that she likes. If you seek and obtain pleasure much of the time despite your fatigue and other symptoms, depression is not at the heart of your problem.

But what if Susan had succumbed to depression *because* of her physical illness? How could one tell whether she felt depressed because of her physical illness or physically ill because she was depressed? The best way is to cure the physical illness and see if the depression clears. However, if the physical illness persists (or if no physical illness is found), treating the depression directly gives the best chance of improving the quality of life.

Another way doctors often use to diagnose depression is a standardized pencil-and-paper quiz such as the Beck Depression Inventory. This self-assessment test can be found in Dr. David Burns' *Feeling Good* (New American Library, 1980). Such tests are helpful but are not infallible. For example, they may fail to detect subtle depression in persons who are not in touch with their feelings.

The traditional and most valuable method of uncovering depression is discussing your situation with a mental health counselor. In two to four sessions you can usually decide if depression or other mental illness is present in sufficient degree to contribute to your fatigue. This process of judging is called a psychological evaluation, a critical step that should not be skipped.

A psychological evaluation allows you to test your feelings and ideas. Are your perceptions accurate? Do your reactions to situations work for or against your best interests? Issues that are more significant than you had previously appreciated may surface. Is your current distress an isolated episode or part of a lifetime pattern? Is it triggered by events in your life, by changes in your needs and desires, or by independent biochemical events? Is psychological treatment likely to help? Is it optional or essential? Is it urgent? People who play down their emotional reactions are especially likely to benefit from the getting-in-touch process that occurs during a psychological evaluation.

Whom should you see for the evaluation? I recommend, first, a visit to your personal physician. Your doctor should know you as a person, care about you, and hold a degree of confidence and comfort that should make it easy to discuss your personal concerns. He will also know the psychiatrists and psychologists in your community. He can thus recommend one who is skilled in treating your condition and is likely to relate well to you. Your physician will also help rule out physical disorders that can cause fatigue and depression. However, do not defer your psychological evaluation until every last physical possibility has been excluded. It is important that both physical and psychological exams be coordinated.

Family physicians and internists also have limitations. A common error is underdiagnosing depression and minimizing the importance of its symptoms. Along with our patients, we tend to assume that emotional distress is due mainly to current life situations or stresses, and we may miss the underlying depressive illness that is making us vulnerable.

Another problem is that we often do not appreciate the episodic nature of fatigue and related symptoms of depression. People prone to depression tend to suffer for months, improve for a long period, then relapse. Physicians who are extremely good at treating individual episodes of depression sometimes slack off as improvement occurs, missing the golden opportunity to work on the longer-term issues that might prevent a relapse.

The psychiatrist is usually most qualified to judge whether depression is present and to suggest the best way to treat it. A psychiatrist has extensive training in doing evaluations. Not all Ph.D. psychologists are equally skilled in the evaluation process. Usually a *general* psychiatrist is better than one whose practice is limited to a single approach such as psychoanalysis or family therapy. The priority at this point is understanding your problem; therefore, you deserve a review with a broad perspective and a wide range of options for treatment.

You should state explicitly that your purpose is an evaluation, to learn whether something is wrong psychologically, if it should be treated, and how? You are not committing to a long series of treatments. Since an evaluation should take only a few visits, the higher cost of a psychiatrist is less important than the quality of the opinion.

If you later decide to enter psychotherapy, you might continue with that psychiatrist or ask for a referral to another psychiatrist, psychologist, psychiatric social worker, or pastoral counselor whose skills or personal characteristics are suited to your needs. Although the psychiatrist's training in evaluation is superior, the ability to counsel effectively depends more on personality: the counselor's, the patient's, and the chemistry between them. A counselor who is not a psychiatrist might well be first choice for treatment. In that case the evaluating psychiatrist should share his evaluation with the treating therapist. The psychiatrist might continue to advise as your treatment progresses, particularly if you require medication, which a nonphysician therapist is not licensed to employ.

The main disadvantage of treatment by a psychiatrist is the cost, which in New Jersey runs about $100 for a forty-five to sixty-minute session. Psychologists and psychiatric social workers charge between $60 and $80.

Special Questions and Answers

Since almost everyone at some time feels "depressed," I have assembled some questions people often ask in considering whether their fatigue could relate to an actual depression or to a passing mood or simply a low-key temperament.

Q: Don't we all have psychological and practical problems that get us down? How can a psychiatrist tell if these are causing my fatigue?

A: Everyone has emotional conflicts to some degree. Usually these are not so severe that they cause depression or chronic fatigue. Our interests and energy levels overcome these drags on our spirits. A psychiatrist can help determine how important these conflicts are. Of course, it's not just the psychiatrist's opinion that counts. Ultimately you will have to judge whether there is a problem worth treating.

Q: I have some of the symptoms of depression, but my family loves me. I am financially secure. There's no reason why I should feel sad. Is depression still a possibility?

A: Yes. Some people who appear to be depressed "for no reason" have psychological issues affecting them of which they are only partly aware. And depression can run in families, so there may be a biological, inherited component. You don't necessarily need a reason to be depressed. It can just happen. Depression is linked to changes in the brain's chemical metabolism. Probably these changes can be caused by various factors that include emotional conflict, physical illnesses, medicines, and other reasons yet unknown.

Q: Are there biochemical tests to diagnose depression?

A: In recent years psychiatry researchers have identified several biochemical tests that distinguish some people with depression from most well people. However, many depressed persons score normal and some well persons score abnormal. Therefore, while biochemical testing is an important research field and has some practical uses, it is not yet good enough for routine use to detect depression.

Q: If I feel depressed sometimes, but am tired all the time, can depression still be the cause?

A: Yes. Certain individuals seem to have a chronic low-grade depression with occasional worsening. Psychiatrists call this pattern a dysphoric personality. Such people tend to be tired much of the time even when they are not extremely depressed. Also, depression can get you into a rut. You may have developed pessimistic habits of thinking and acting so that activities lose their appeal. Thus a habit of tiredness persists even after the general depression abates.

Q: What if I have energetic periods between my tiredness and depression?

A: Cyclical ups and downs are characteristic of a very special form of depression called manic-depressive illness. Periods of fatigue and depression alternate with times of powerful enthusiasm and energy. Recognizing the manic-depressive pattern is extremely important, since the standard antidepression medicines usually do not work. However, supplements containing the mineral lithium are usually extremely effective.

Q: Is there a relationship among fatigue, depression, and senility?

A: Indeed, depression in older persons is often mistaken for senility. It may require a detailed neurological and psychological evaluation to know which is which. Any time an older person appears to be losing mental power, a physician should search for treatable physical and mental causes. Depression causing loss of concentration and slowed thinking as well as fatigue is one of the disorders most frequently misdiagnosed as senility.

Q: Is overuse of alcohol or drugs a sign of depression?

A: Depression can be the underlying problem that causes excessive use of alcohol or other mood-altering drugs. Or the drugs themselves can be the cause of depression. Either way, excessive use of alcohol or other drugs should be a red flag to look for depression.

Q: Can the combination of depression and fatigue create special risk for suicide?

A: A suicidally depressed person who is profoundly tired might lack the initiative or drive to act on the suicidal thoughts. However, a particularly dangerous time for such individuals is when they begin to recover their energy. A major disappointment may revive suicidal impulses while the energy to act remains strong. Occasional fleeting thoughts about suicide are common and, usually lead only to the recognition that one is depressed. However, frequent or prolonged thoughts of suicide, especially if one thinks of specific methods, should sound an alarm. Seek competent care immediately.

Q: If I am tired from a physical illness, isn't it natural to become discouraged? Won't the psychiatrist blame my emotions instead of the physical illness that is really the cause?

A: Excellent questions. Almost everyone who is chronically ill from a physical illness becomes discouraged to a degree, often sufficiently to trigger a genuine depression. That is why it's wise to see your regular physician to check on your physical status. Often one needs to treat both the physical illness and the depression.

Or you might be depressed and fatigued by a physical illness that has not yet been diagnosed. If you've had no previous problem with depression and psychiatric evaluation reveals no conflicts likely to produce depression, your physician should be especially careful to search for diseases that can cause or mimic depression. Even with a history of previous depression or current emotional conflicts, your physician should check for physical causes.

Q: Is it common for unnoticed physical conditions to contribute to depression?

A: Probably so, according to Dr. David Sternberg of the Yale School of Medicine, who specifically examined this issue. In one study of patients diagnosed as psychiatrically ill, a physical illness was the main cause in 8 percent, and an exacerbating factor in more than a fifth. Almost half of these physical conditions had been undiagnosed previously. Although some were conditions that are difficult to diagnose, often the failure to detect them was because no one had looked carefully for physical factors. In one study, Dr. Sternberg notes, a third of practicing psychiatrists stated that they felt incompetent to perform a rudimentary physical examination and two-thirds stated that they rarely if ever do so.

Q: Which are the main physical causes of depression?

A: Any disease can produce depression indirectly by causing discomfort, worry, or fear. Certain diseases produce depression directly, probably by affecting the metabolism of the brain. In these cases depression is part of the physical illness, not just an emotional reaction to it.

Medications are among the most common physical causes of depression. Many of the drugs listed in Appendix 6 as causing chronic fatigue also can precipitate depression. The most important of these include the anti-high blood pressure drugs clonidine, reserpine, methyldopa, and the beta blockers. Others include birth control pills, tranquilizers, antiulcer drugs, anti-inflammatory pain medicines, diet pills, and the increasingly popular calcium channel-blocking agents. If you take medicines regularly consult Appendix 6 or look them up in the drug references provided in Chapter 13.

Depression can result from endocrine disorders, including underactive thyroid, adrenal gland disease, diabetes, and abnormalities of mineral metabolism. Wilson's disease, a rare abnormality of copper metabolism, can trigger depression and other personality changes. Deficiency or malabsorption of vitamins B_{12}, B_1, B_3, and B_6 can cause depression and fatigue.

Chronic viral illness such as hepatitis, Epstein-Barr virus syndrome, and AIDS can trigger depression, as can the later stages of the still-important bacterial infection syphilis. Autoimmune inflammatory conditions such as rheumatoid arthritis and the less common but even more disabling systemic lupus erythematosus can bring out depression. Neurological diseases that can trigger depression include Alzheimer's disease (premature senility), strokes, seizure disorders, brain tumors, and Parkinson's disease.

Certain cancers, especially cancer of the pancreas or cancer of the bowel may cause depression and fatigue as the first noticeable sign. Researchers speculate this might result from the cancer's effect on the immune system or from hormones that a cancer might produce. Occupational or environmental pollutants such as mercury, lead, solvents, or pesticides can also be the cause of depression. Fortunately almost all these conditions can be identified or suspected after a thorough review of the medical history, physical exam, standard blood tests, and perhaps a brain-wave test (EEG).

Probably there are other physical causes of depression that have not yet been identified. Indeed, most depression may be the result of unidentified biochemical events. However, regardless of the cause, the gratifying fact is that current treatments for depression are usually effective.

Q: Can one have both depression and anxiety?

A: Yes. As discussed in Chapter 6, anxiety can lead to depression. On the other hand, depression can also trigger anxiety. It is important to decide which is the main problem because the best medicines for each are different. Tranquilizers, which are excellent for anxiety, do not help depression and can make it worse.

Q: What are the treatments for depression?

A: There are various kinds of talk therapy. Interpersonal psychotherapy assumes that depression is rooted in relationships with other people and that improving patterns of interaction will help the depression. Cognitive therapy assumes that depression is based on unrealistically negative views and habits of thought that people have about themselves, their world, and their future. Improvement should come by reevaluating one's situation, and by adjusting one's attitudes. Analytic psychotherapy, related to but less intense than psychoanalysis, holds that vulnerability to depression lies mainly in one's childhood personality development and its symbolic, usually unconscious, replay in one's current life.

These and other psychotherapy approaches can be effective. However, the most important factor in a person's benefiting from psychotherapy is not the type of therapy but the quality of the relationship that develops between patient and therapist. You do not have to like the therapist, but you must "connect" or relate to each other at a gut or emotional level. The personal chemistry is a critical element. If after a few months you are not feeling better and feel poorly related to the therapist, you should discuss this directly with him or her, reevaluate your situation and consider asking for a referral to another counselor. However, if you have tried several therapists and none has seemed right, ask yourself candidly if you might be resisting forming the relationship you need to benefit from treatment.

Antidepressant medicines can also help depression, usually within a few weeks. Medicines are particularly important for depression where there is no "good reason" to feel bad. Antidepressant medicines probably work by altering the chemistry of the brain. They are relatively safe and effective when properly monitored. It is now practical to measure the actual blood levels of most antidepressant drugs. This helps to fine-tune dosage to obtain maximum benefit with less risk of side effects.

The few studies that have compared the effectiveness of drug therapy to talk therapy suggest that, on the average, they are about equally effective. This result may be deceptive, however, since certain individuals probably respond better to medication and others to talk. For many, optimum treatment probably includes drug treatment for three to six months at the same time as talk therapy.

Other drastic treatments such as electroshock therapy are reserved for serious cases that do not respond to medicines or talk.

CHAPTER

9

SLEEP PROBLEMS

This chapter tackles the important question of when you should suspect that poor sleep contributes to your fatigue. No one knows why nature requires that humans sleep. One research scientist remarked, only half in jest, that sleep is nature's way of keeping us from roaming in the dark and bumping into things. If so, the allure of sleep was dealt a blow when Thomas A. Edison invented the electric light and Steve Allen hit late-night television. In fact, modern school children reported a full hour's less sleep each day than did children surveyed in 1900. Undersleeping is a way of life for many busy Americans.

There is no simple test to measure whether you are getting enough sleep: we have to look at indirect indicators. For example, two-thirds of American adults sleep between seven and eight hours per night. One-fifth sleep fewer than six hours and one tenth sleep more than nine. Therefore, suspect you sleep too little if you usually sleep much less than average—six hours or less on most nights.

Of course, some individuals who sleep seven or eight hours would feel better with more. A few rare souls do well with four hours. Number of hours slept is a useful but imperfect guide for deciding if you are "short" of sleep.

Another indicator is a change in sleeping pattern. If you are tired and getting forty-five minutes less sleep than in the past, you are probably getting too little rest. Compare sleep now to the amount you got when you last felt well. If you think you've "always" been tired, think way back to when you felt well—in high school, on your first job, on a long vacation.

A third clue that you might be short of sleep is the presence of factors that might increase your need for sleep. Athletes often feel they need more sleep when in heavy training. Sustained mental work or emotional stress can increase the amount of sleep needed to feel well. Sleep disrupted by physical pain and emotional distress can increase your sleep needs.

Other clues that too little sleep may be a problem include:

Intense grogginess on awakening. Few working people wake up without an alarm and feeling well. So don't worry if you hate your first fifteen minutes awake. However, if you are not alert and feeling well by the time you dress, consider too little sleep as a possible cause.

"I can't wake up until I've had my coffee." The problem may be caffeine addiction, but simple lack of sleep can also be the cause.

Weekend sleeping. Sleeping until noon on weekends and holidays often means you haven't been getting the sleep you need during the week.

Nodding off. Do you "drop off" easily at plays, concerts, or management meetings? It could be boredom, but also suspect either poor quality or not enough sleep.

Frantic pace. If your life is incredibly busy and you haven't time to pause, your pace of living may be wearing you out. Insufficient sleep plus overload equals fatigue.

If you suspect *not enough sleep* is part of your problem, commit yourself to a prescription of more sleep. Increase your nightly sleep time by forty-five minutes for two weeks. See if you feel better. If you have difficulty falling asleep earlier or can't wake up later, ask your physician to consider a brief trial of a mild sleeping medicine to help you "reset" your personal clock for an earlier bedtime. A useful alternative might be an afternoon nap.

You can make an enlightened decision about how much sleep is best for you.

Insomnia

Millions of Americans *know* they do not get enough sleep—and not because they love late-night TV. They can't fall asleep. Others wake at 3:00 A.M and can't go back to sleep. They suffer from insomnia, that agony of night which next day leaves its mark in sleepiness and fatigue.

National surveys find a third of adult Americans have some problem with insomnia. At least 15 percent of us consider our insomnia serious and chronic.

Do you really have insomnia? Most of us have occasional difficulty falling or staying asleep. An exciting or troublesome situation in our lives, a change in sleeping location, illness, jet lag, or altered sleep schedule may induce a restless night or two. Don't be concerned about these. However, if you can't sleep for one or two nights every week, you have moderate insomnia. If you suffer three nights a week or more, your problem is certainly serious enough to do something about.

Thirty minutes or more to fall asleep should be considered abnormal. Reawakening during the night for thirty minutes or more is also abnormal, although, waking during the night is not abnormal in itself. In fact, most adults wake momentarily fifteen or twenty times each night without remembering it and without ill effects. One or two short episodes, for example a trip to the bathroom, should not affect how you feel the next day. Five or more *remembered* wakings during a night is abnormal.

Some individuals think they have insomnia but don't. They are alert and feel well after only six hours sleep but lie awake for two hours each night thinking they should sleep for eight hours. They become bored, frustrated, and fear they'll pay health consequences for not sleeping enough. Their worry and expectation of trouble *is* fatiguing. Such people are victims of their mistaken belief about how much sleep they need. The cure is simple: go to bed later or get up earlier—and *find something rewarding to do with the extra hours gained.*

The following factors are most often responsible for genuine insomnia:

Biology. Some insomniacs may be biologically different from good sleepers. Poor sleepers tend to be chronically sensitive, hyper-alert, and easily awakened. They have more rapid heart rates and higher body temperatures than good sleepers do. They are particularly vulnerable to ordinary environmental intrusions—someone else going to the bathroom, a truck passing by—or the disrupting effects of emotional stress. Concern about the adequacy of sleep could create a vicious cycle of more worry/less sleep/less energy/increased concern.

Illness. Many illnesses cause discomfort that reduces the restfulness of sleep and promotes insomnia. Examples appear in Table 9.1. Treating these conditions should lead to better sleep. Ironically, better sleep may reduce the severity of the disease symptoms. Such feedback loops are very common among conditions that affect the mind/body interface. If you suspect a medical condition might be affecting your sleep, discuss the situation with your doctor.

Emotional/mental arousal often leads to physical arousal, destroying the inner tranquility essential for sleep. For example, anxiety promotes insomnia (and insomnia makes anxiety worse). Happy and interesting

Table 9.1: MEDICAL CONDITIONS THAT AFFECT SLEEP

Condition	*Typical Symptom*	*Self-treatment*
Angina	Tightness, pain, or pressure in chest, arm, or jaw	Discuss with doctor; go to emergency room promptly if severe or prolonged
Arthritis	Aches and pains	Pain medicine*
Asthma	Wheezing, cough	Asthma medicines**
Bronchitis, emphysema	Cough, mucus, shortness of breath	Discuss with doctor; possibly oxygen
Epilepsy	Seizures	Some persons have seizures only during sleep; bedmate should observe
Esophagus irritation or reflux	Heartburn, belching, chest distress	Elevate head of bed; antacids; no food after dinner. *Careful!* Angina can mimic esophagus pain
Gallstones	Right upper abdominal or back pain	Discuss with doctor
Headache	Headache	Pain medicine*; discuss with doctor
Heart failure	Shortness of breath, cough	Elevate head of bed; discuss with doctor
Hypoglycemia	Anxiety, hunger	Discuss with doctor
Nasal	Nose stuffed, cough, mucus, dry mouth	Decongestants, antihistamines, nose drops
Thyroid	Feel "hyper" or "hypo"	Discuss with doctor
Tooth-grinding	Jaw aches in A.M.	Discuss with dentist; sometimes stress-related
Ulcers	Stomach or back pain, nausea	Antacids; discuss with doctor
Urinary diseases	Frequent urination	Discuss with doctor; no fluids after 6 P.M.; many potential causes

* Choose non-narcotic pain medicines that do not contain caffeine.

** Most asthma medicines are stimulants.

thoughts can also hamper sleep. For example, wakened at 3:00 A.M by my young daughter, I start to think about the article I am writing and become too alert to return to sleep.

Depression. Most depressed people fall asleep easily but wake extra early—often ruminating about their distress and unable to recapture sleep. They feel fatigued throughout the day. However, other depressed people actually sleep longer than usual, perhaps an escape from sadness or a reflection of their lack of interest in life's activities. This sleep tends not to be restful and daytime tiredness remains a problem. Many depressed persons focus exclusively on their fatigue and sleep problems, perhaps to avoid dealing with their sadness or anger. Some people become so upset about their insomnia as to cause depression or anxiety states. Often one cannot be sure whether the sleep problem or the depression came first. Often both need to be treated. Good sleep is as fragile as a porcelain egg. Any distress—physical or emotional—can break it.

Drugs that disrupt or improve sleep. The two drugs that most often disturb sleep are caffeine and alcohol. In sensitive individuals even one evening drink of coffee or alcohol can upset sleep.

Ironically, the prescription drugs that most often disturb sleep are tranquilizers and sleeping pills. The most popular are benzodiazepine-type chemicals. These include Dalmane, Restoril, Valium, Librium, Tranxene, Ativan, and Halcion.

Benzodiazepines are safer than the barbiturates that were the previously most favored type of sedative (for example Seconal, Phenobarbital). However, benzodiazepines can be habit-forming. If you take them regularly they become less effective, and you may need to increase the dose to maintain their usefulness. Benzodiazepines can distort the normal cycle of sleeping and dreaming. Whether this effect is harmful is still unclear.

Long-acting benzodiazepines such as Dalmane may produce drowsiness the next day. Anxious individuals often prefer this daytime sedation, others will not. Halcion is a short-acting benzodiazepine that does not sedate the next day. However, some suffer a rebound wake-up as Halcion becomes inactive during the wee hours of the morning. Restoril provides an intermediate duration of activity.

After frequent use, all benzodiazepines (and barbiturates) can induce withdrawal symptoms when they are stopped. Over all, the benzodiazepine sedatives are extremely valuable for occasional insomnia, but frequent use can perpetuate one's sleep problems.

If you take sleeping pills regularly, don't stop suddenly. Talk with your physician to plot a withdrawal strategy. Many people experience little or no withdrawal symptoms. Others take several nights to a month to adjust. The good news is that many chronic sedative-takers actually sleep *better* once they've gotten off the pills.

Other sleeping medicines. A low dose of a prescription tricylcic antidepressant (such as Elavil, Sinequan, Norpramin) taken before bedtime sedates and often improves sleep quality. This effect occurs the first night, in contrast to the antidepressant effect, which usually takes several weeks. Because these drugs are long-acting, many individuals complain of grogginess the next day.

Except for Seldane, all the currently available antihistamines are sedating. Taken before bed (without a stimulating decongestant!), they make fairly effective sleeping pills. Sleeping pills that are available without prescription usually contain antihistamines.

L-tryptophan, an amino acid available from health food stores, has a mild sedative effect. Research studies using l-2-gram doses suggest that tryptophan's sleep-promoting effect is modest but real. In my experience, only 20 percent of those who try tryptophan find it fully satisfactory. We know little about possible long-term side effects from prolonged use.

A few individuals find *aspirin* an effective sleeping aid, but don't take aspirin if you are vulnerable to ulcers or gastritis, since it can make these conditions worse.

Environment. A comfortable environment supports good sleep. A distracting, uncomfortable, or threatening one makes good sleep impossible. Among factors you should consider in evaluating your sleep environment are noise, light, temperature, humidity, and physical security.

Habits and body rhythm. The human body is a creature of cycles and habits. Most individuals are more receptive to sleep at particular times, reflecting rhythms that are partly biological and partly psychological.

Normal persons undergo ninty-minute cycles of increased and decreased alertness throughout the day. There are similar but not identical cycles during sleep—dreaming, body-temperature change, rapid eye movements, genital organ excitement. Alertness is linked to body-temperature cycles. We feel more alert when body temperature is higher and sluggish when body temperature falls. The sleep/wake cycle and the body-temperature cycle can adjust to changed sleep schedules—although a time lag is required to get back "in phase." Therefore *irregular sleeping habits tend to disrupt the ability to sleep well.*

Unfortunately, many individuals vary their bedtimes considerably. The most common pattern is delayed bedtime and late rising on weekends, causing miserable Mondays. Shift work is particularly destructive. As a medical resident at New York's Mount Sinai Hospital, I changed work shifts every five days. Just as I began to get used to one sleep pattern, we would shift again. Misery. Most sleep experts believe that shift work increases both physical and mental ills. Jet lag creates similar problems. Unnaturally rapid changes in biological rhythms can take a terrible toll.

The bottom line for sleep is that regularity pays—by capitalizing on helpful biological rhythms and by creating the psychological expectation that sleep will indeed arrive. Familiar presleep rituals such as reading, a glass of milk, or tooth-brushing condition us to accept the sleep that follows.

Unfortunately, the sword of expectation cuts both ways. For example, during a bout of temporary emotional distress a few nights of poor sleep could create anxiety about future insomnia. Then the person lies awake, vigilantly watching for sleep to approach—which of course prevents it. A self-fulfilling expectation is created. Sleep clinics are full of once-normal sleepers who failed to recover their usual rhythm after a temporary disruption. Treatment requires breaking the counterproductive expectations to form new expectations and habits that promote sleep.

Disrupted body rhythm is responsible for a common sleep problem called delayed-phase sleep syndrome. Biologically we tend to run in twenty-five-hour-day cycles which we must modify to fit into a twenty-four-hour day. If guided by our tiredness, most of us would go to sleep an hour later each day—which is what happens on weekends. But jobs and family do not permit this during the work week. Many of us therefore drift into a later bedtime while still having to get up early. The result is chronic daytime fatigue *and* "insomnia" if we try to sleep earlier.

For a few individuals ("night owls") the natural tendency toward later bedtimes is exaggerated by an inclination toward late-night vitality and early-morning sluggishness. In contrast, "larks" are individuals who are full of enthusiasm in the morning but tire early at night. Larks and owls can adapt to necessity, but not always without pain.

The key to recognizing that "insomnia" results from the delayed-phase sleep syndrome is that you can sleep well if you follow your inclinations to stay up very late at night and wake up late as well. To get on a schedule to be at work at 9:00 A.M., such people must "reset" their biological clock. One way to do this is to stay awake later and later each night (until 5:00 A.M. rather than 2:00 A.M.), rising eight hours later until you hit the bedtime and wake-up time you desire. Then *stick to that schedule.* Don't start staying up late again. That way you'll kick your "insomnia" and cure your daytime fatigue. Another way may be through bright-light exposure for several hours in the morning. Known as chronotherapy, such techniques for cycle shifting should be supervised by a physician, preferably one trained in sleep problems.

Gaining a Good Night's Sleep

The following principles serve to cure or prevent insomnia. You can try them on your own or in consultation with your family physician or perhaps a psychologist.

1. Figure out how much sleep you really need to feel your best. If you require two alarm clocks to wake up and you fight sleepiness much of the day, add forty-five minutes to your nighttime sleep or get a *regular* short nap. After two to four weeks, judge the results.

2. Become a creature of habit. Go to bed and wake up at the same time every day, seven days a week, for at least one month. If you do stay up late or have a bad night's sleep, still get up near your usual hour. Stay awake until near your regular bedtime that night, even if you feel exhausted.

3. The regular-bedtime rule can sometimes be broken if you are not tired at bedtime. Trying to force sleep can create frustrations and negative conditioning that hampers future sleep. If you are *never* tired at bedtime and wake up feeling well, you may actually require less sleep than you think. If you are never tired at bedtime but are always tired the next morning, you may be an out-of-phase "owl." If so, consultation with a sleep specialist is in order.

4. If you waken at night and don't fall back to sleep immediately, relax, listen to music, read. If you feel frustrated, leave the bedroom and do a quiet activity until you feel sleepy again.

5. Take a caffeine- and alcohol-free holiday. Avoid large late-evening meals that might upset your stomach, but do not go to bed hungry. High-carbohydrate and high-fat foods as an evening snack tend to promote sedation. Avoid chocolate—it's a stimulant.

6. Exercise can allay depression and anxiety. This promotes better sleep. Think of it as burning up the nervous energy that keeps you awake at night. But avoid exercise just before bedtime; it may tend to keep you awake.

7. Relax in the evening as you stage down toward sleep. Muscle relaxation, deep-breathing exercises, meditation, imagining pleasant scenes—all enhance relaxation. Do these at least an hour or two before sleep, since these exercises also invigorate and may keep you awake. Light reading or pleasant nonvocal music may help. Making these staging-down activities a ritual will reinforce them as conditioners preceding your transition to sleep.

8. Rid yourself of unpleasant thoughts, worries, and uncertainties. Keep a diary and "spill it out" if that helps. Leave your worries and plans for tomorrow on the paper, where they will be safe and no longer a burden on your mind.

9. Let the bedroom be your oasis of comfort. Set the temperature, humidity, and noise level to your wishes. If external noise is a problem, consider a masking background noise (music, an electric fan) or earplugs. Block out street light. Obviously, you deserve a comfortable bed.

10. Use your bedroom for sex or sleeping *only*. Do not review bills in bed. Do not discuss hectic issues with your bedmate. Do not watch exciting crime shows before sleep.

11. You may use sleeping pills occasionally, if prescribed by your doctor. For mild sedation I prefer simple antihistamines. For frequent use I prefer low-dose tricyclic antidepressants or the benzodiazepines. Discuss all medication issues with your doctor.

12. Are you suffering from stress overload? Do things sometimes feel more than you can manage? Is there constant strain? Discuss it with your doctor and read Chapter 6. Could you be depressed? Do you become self-critical? Angry? Feel helpless? Apathetic? Again, talk with your doctor and read about it in Chapter 8. Anxiety and depression can ruin sleep and create fatigue.

Other Sleep Disorders

Sleep Apnea. *Apnea* means cessation of breathing. Many individuals occasionally stop breathing while asleep for ten seconds or more. Certain individuals—perhaps 1 percent or more of the adult population—stop breathing many times, awaken partially or fully, and thereby suffer unsatisfying sleep and sleepiness throughout the next day.

There are two main kinds of sleep apnea: obstructive (in which collapse of the upper airways during sleep prevents good breathing) and the less common central kind (in which the diaphragm and chest muscles "forget" to breathe). An individual can have both conditions.

Obstructive sleep apnea should be considered for anyone who snores frequently and is usually tired during the day. These symptoms may be unrelated to apnea, but a substantial number of chronically tired snorers do have obstructive sleep apnea.

The victims of obstructive sleep apnea may not recognize their difficulty breathing or their brief awakenings. However, they find sleep unsatisfying, and tiredness plagues them much of the day. Sleep apnea can also cause a wide range of problems in addition to fatigue: deterioration of intellectual capacity and judgment, loss of sexual interest, emotional instability and personality changes, headaches that are usually worse in the morning or after a nap, certain forms of heart and lung disease, and possibly high blood pressure and stroke. Advanced cases may have blackouts during the day or episodes of zombielike behavior, sleepwalking, bed-wetting, or hallucinations—as if one were dreaming awake.

The personality changes of sleep apnea should not be passed over as psychological or as "normal" senility. I repeat, if you are frequently tired and usually snore, suspect the possibility of obstructive sleep apnea. While obstructive sleep apnea can occur at any age, be especially concerned if you are sixty or older, are obese, have chronic lung or heart disease, or have high blood pressure or a history of stroke.

Ask someone to observe your sleep, ideally for at least two hours. The observer can read with a dim light or even watch TV, since the loud snoring serves as an easy marker for breathing. The observer should look for changes in the pattern and loudness of snoring, recurring pauses in breathing of ten seconds or more, and such signs of distress as gurgling in the throat or unsettling body movements. (Sleep experts recommend recording the breath sounds on a tape recorder and playing it for your doctor. Frankly, I have never been able to record clearly enough to make this method work.)

If you are suspicious that nighttime breathing may be difficult, discuss it with your doctor, but also strongly consider seeking advice from a specialist in sleep disorders. Most of us in family medicine, internal medicine, and pediatrics are not yet well trained in the diagnosis of serious sleep disorders. An overnight stay in a sleep laboratory may not be necessary, since there are now apnea monitors that can monitor your breathing pattern at home while you sleep.

Central sleep apnea. Victims of central sleep apnea often do not snore. The problem here is that the brain "forgets" to signal the chest and diaphragm muscles to breathe. As a result, the same complications may develop as in obstructive sleep apnea. However, people with central sleep apnea usually will realize that they are waking many times during the night. They may complain of insomnia or poor sleep. Individuals with emphysema and chronic lung diseases may develop a similar illness. Sleeping pills do not help and may make these conditions worse. Observation while sleeping is important to detect central sleep apnea, but this should be done by an expert, preferably in a sleep laboratory, since snoring is not present to signal breathing interruptions.

Consider the possibility of central sleep apnea if you are chronically tired and wake frequently through the night, feel restless during the night, or awaken gasping for breath.

Leg movements at night. Millions are afflicted with a condition that sleep specialists call periodic leg movements, or nocturnal myoclonus. Perhaps as many as a third of people over sixty-five suffer from this problem.

Small or large contractions of the leg muscles occur in bursts every fifteen to thirty seconds for minutes or hours every night. These contractions can reduce the effectiveness of sleep or trigger hundreds of brief awakenings. The sleeping individual is almost never aware of the leg movements, although a bed partner might report that kicking or unusual activity occurs. Instead, the victim of periodic leg movements complains of unsatisfying sleep, frequent awakening, or tiredness.

A few who have periodic leg movements also have a daytime syndrome known as restless legs. They feel a need to move their legs repeatedly. A nervous feeling within the legs is relieved by movement. Benzodiazepine sleeping pills seem to help this problem. Tricylic antidepressant pills may make it worse.

Although you may suspect you suffer from periodic leg movements based on testimony from an observer at home (or from the disarray of your bedding), confirmation should be obtained by observation in a sleep laboratory.

Can you be tired because you sleep too much? Yes. Overlong sleeping or napping can leave you feeling chronically sluggish. The irony is that people who lack energy or feel unalert may try to solve the problem with even more sleep. Sometimes sleeping too much is a sign that something else is wrong. Many depressed people feel more energetic when they are forced to wake up several hours earlier than usual. If you might be sleeping too much, try waking up thirty minutes earlier for two weeks to do something that you enjoy.

Narcolepsy. Narcolepsy is truly a sleeping sickness that affects perhaps a quarter of a million Americans. Experts estimate that perhaps half of those with narcolepsy remain undiagnosed. Since medical treatment is fairly effective, the failure to diagnose this sleep disorder can cause decades of unnecessary suffering.

The main symptom of narcolepsy is uncontrolled sleepiness. Narcoleptics fall asleep easily in boring settings such as lectures or while watching television. However, they also may drop off at work, while driving or eating, or during other normal activities. Unlike others for whom sleepiness and alertness ebb and flow, narcoleptics are sleepy almost all the time. The narcoleptic benefits from sleeping but just cannot get enough.

Narcoleptics may experience other peculiar symptoms, such as sudden attacks of muscle weakness called cataplexy. Some narcoleptics have visual hallucinations, like a dream while awake. Sometimes minutes or hours pass with no memory of what has transpired. Narcolepsy should be considered possible when there is substantial and long-standing daytime sleepiness. If spells of muscle weakness or daytime hallucinations also occur, narcolepsy is probable. However, disabling sleepiness is often narcolepsy's only symptom.

A simple test for narcolepsy that does not require a full sleep-laboratory examination is called the multiple sleep latency test. Persons suspected of narcolepsy are allowed several opportunities to sleep at two-hour intervals during the day. Narcoleptics average only four minutes before the onset of sleep (normal persons typically take about ten minutes). If you suspect narcolepsy, consultation with a sleep specialist is mandatory.

Narcolepsy is treated with a combination of special schedule planning and medicines that stimulate wakefulness. For many, the difference is dramatic, returning disabled narcoleptics to reasonably normal and productive lives.

When to Consult a Sleep Specialist

Most people with mild-to-moderate sleep problems can benefit from the simple advice contained here. Your family physician can help you adapt such advice to your personal situation. If this does not work, or if your problem is severe or long-standing, you might do better by consulting a specialist in sleep problems.

Sleep study as a medical specialty commanded almost no interest before the 1970s. The majority of practicing physicians have never attended a course on sleep disorders. Most communities do not have any sleep specialists. Therefore, if one wants state-of-the-art advice it will often be necessary to seek consultation at a medical-school-based sleep disorders center.

See Appendix 7 for a listing of sleep disorder centers in your area. Sleep centers currently exist in about two-thirds of the states, but not all have attained the association's highest rating of "fully accredited." The major problems are that sleep studies often require several nights away from home, they are expensive, and health insurance coverage varies.

CHAPTER

10

SITUATIONAL FATIGUE: THE BODY'S WAY OF SAYING NO

Shakespeare wrote in *A Winter's Tale* that "A merry heart goes all the day—a sad one tires in a mile."

Countless examples in everyday life testify to this truth. I know a surgeon who views his work as the only challenging, meaningful endeavor this world has to offer. Everything else seems trivial. In the operating theater, he is electrified—alert and tireless throughout the longest, most difficult procedures. At other times he is plagued by chronic fatigue, vague aches, and difficulty concentrating. He feels on the verge of collapse during morning medical-staff meetings, even after a full night's sleep. He is too tired to attend social functions, to review the finances of his medical practice, to fill out insurance forms, or even to exchange a few words with his wife. On days off from work, including his rare vacations, he's tired. This man has an extreme case of somaticizing, in which the body physically expresses a mental attitude.

Physicians overdiagnose the tired housewife syndrome. However, the stereotype is based on reality; it is another example of situational fatigue. Daily tasks of vacuuming, laundering, shopping, and endless errands are taxing primarily because they are *drudgery.* They bring no surprises (except unpleasant ones), no gratitude, no reward of creativity. The tiredness they create is not based so much on energy expenditure as on the quality of motivation. Working while the spirit lags is like driving with the brakes locked! You burn all your fuel just to drag along.

In this vein, being "too tired for sex" has been the perennial marital malady. Of course, the individuals aren't too tired in the usual sense. Calorie expenditure for sex relations is not much more than walking up a few flights of stairs. Tell a person who's too tired for sex that a winning lottery ticket is available two flights up and he or she would probably bound from bed to get it in an instant.

Still, the tiredness is absolutely genuine. They are mentally battered from handling many tedious events in the course of a day and are eager to escape in carefree sleep. For many, tiredness would evaporate if the path to the bedroom had been strewn with petals—vital conversation, sharing, good will. They're not tired so much as saturated with negative emotion. They aren't inclined to make a sharp turnaround, whereas a gradual one might have been possible. For other "tired" couples, the problem is more fundamental. They need to work out disagreement, anger, or resentment between them—or to learn to leave such things outside the bedroom door.

Situational fatigue is extraordinarily common. But the cause won't be revealed by blood tests or by the usual medical history. Nonetheless, situational fatigue is a subclinical fact of life. Its victims are not mentally ill. Situational fatigue is not a psychiatric diagnosis, like depression or anxiety. It is nevertheless a very human reaction to the unpleasant or threatening. Fatigue is very often the body's way of saying no.

The key task is to identify when motivational brakes are wearing down your body's engine, since internal resistance of this type is not always recognized.

I urge patients to use their "inner ear" to capture the message their body is transmitting. If your tiredness in certain situations is saying "I dread this" or groaning "I'm bored" or "Not again," repugnance rather than body metabolism may be the cause. The acid test is your reaction to a more pleasant prospect. The energy for tennis but not for a job task is a clue that should make you think. The fatigue triggering turn-off may be *any* negative feeling or emotion, ranging from simple distaste to a threat to self-esteem. You may or may not be aware of why you feel put off. The key is to recognize the feeling, if it is there. Figure out the reason why later.

This litmus test can be used by the chronically tired for all the chores you "haven't the strength" for. Easy ones might be a visit from your mother-in-law, work on your income tax, negotiating with the auto shop over your repair bill. Annoyance, resentment, frustration, fear—all can produce instant "fatigue."

Equally easy to identify are the energizing effects of good news or opportunities. You feel listless, run-down, out of energy when suddenly you receive free tickets to a hockey game, a friend calls to share fascinating gossip, or you're invited to play bridge or poker. Often the excitement of something you want to do erases the fatigue.

More complicated situations might obscure the motivational or situational component, but it can still be heard if you pause to listen carefully.

Randy Pauling was twenty-nine when he sought help because he was always tired. He had married Harriet after a stormy whirlwind courtship. About six months later he became fatigued. He liked his work with the telephone company, but by late afternoon he began to feel worn out. By the end of dinner he was totally depleted. He joked somewhat bitterly that "Not tonight, dear" had become his motto. Sexual frequency decreased toward the vanishing point, much to Harriet's dismay.

Randy didn't understand why he was tired, at least not at first. He was not depressed. Depression has a global effect, diminishing interest in most usual activities. His tiredness seemed somewhat selective: home, evening, sex. Randy and Harriet separated the following year, whereupon Randy's energy returned. Their marriage had been a mismatch. Initial infatuation was powerful, but they had not gotten to know or trust each other well. Fatigue in Randy's case was a way of saying no to emotional intimacy with Harriet as well as "I'm not ready" to acknowledging that their marriage was in trouble. Thus fatigue was a method of avoidance.

Randy's second marriage is a good one. He is more mature, and this relationship seems solid. He looks forward to getting home at night and has little trouble with fatigue. When Randy does become tired for no good reason, which still occurs occasionally, he takes this as a message from himself to himself: something is wrong, somewhere; take a careful look.

Mrs. Dempsey also has situational fatigue. She was fifty-five when her husband died. She had a happy marriage, in which her husband took total responsibility for family finances and record-keeping. Mrs. Dempsey had run the house and worked part time, but she felt unequal to the task of handling the finances. The first year after her husband's death she "prepared" her taxes by bringing all the loose bills and checkbooks she could find to the accountant and leaving them on his desk. The accountant worked out an estimate of what she owed but told her that next year she'd have to organize her records before he could make sense of them. Mrs. Dempsey felt defeated. Just finding her bills and checkbooks had been a tremendous effort. It had taken days of fatiguing procrastination just to start her search. Next year, she feared, it would all be much worse.

Each month's bill-paying and check-balancing became more of an ordeal. She had never been well organized, but now it took hours to complete just two or three checks. She became tired just thinking about it and could barely summon the energy to work on the task for more than twenty minutes at a time. The following April she just stared at the stacks of papers on her desk. As her fatigue increased, she decided to skip her appointment with the accountant that year. She didn't file a tax return. Her income wasn't very high, she thought. She'd wait until her energy returned. Of course it didn't.

Mrs. Dempsey is now three years behind in filing tax returns. She rarely works on her financial records. But she thinks about them a lot, keeps promising herself new starts, and feels increasingly guilty about having let things slide so far. Her tiredness is now pervasive and she can't concentrate on anything for long. There just isn't "time" to get things done.

Mrs. Dempsey saw a psychotherapist. She discovered an unresolved mourning for her husband and a lifelong self-confidence problem that had hardly bothered her so long as her husband took care of the "difficult" tasks. Her phobia about record-keeping was analyzed as a reluctance to accept responsibility for herself or to give up her wish to be taken care of. Perhaps she is clinging to a magical belief that by not taking charge a white knight (or husband) will show up to save her.

Unfortunately, these psychotherapy insights did not set things right. Bills continued to accumulate and her blank tax returns sit in a bottom drawer. Clearly something more was needed to break through the cycle of procrastination and fatigue. I recommended a fresh start: a new accountant who would sit down with Mrs. Dempsey and her financial papers, pull them together, and plead for mercy from the IRS. After that he'd train Mrs. Dempsey to do the books herself or, if that failed, hire her a bookkeeper to make a "house call" once a month. I hoped that once bill-paying and record-keeping had become routine they would lose their forbidding power and fatigue would not prevail.

I'd like to report a happy ending, but, Mrs. Dempsey still feels trapped by her predicament. She's unwilling to follow through on any plan. She sees her fatigue as stemming from her tax and record-keeping problems but blames her procrastination in dealing with them on her fatigue. She is ensnared by this vicious cycle and has not yet summoned the energy to break free.

Boredom or dislike of work may be the most common source of situational fatigue. Jane Miller, twenty-four, works for her father's small manufacturing company. She intends to take over its management in the distant future and has already made her mark as the company's top sales person. She has been almost continuously tired for three months. This began a month after she was taken off sales and assigned the job of bookkeeper. This was to be a temporary position as part of her training. However, as the months go by she strongly suspects that she will not be allowed to get back to sales or to move on to learn the manufacturing end of the company's business.

Jane enjoyed sales, especially the contact with people. She finds accounting dull and isolating and views the job change as a demotion. Fatigue is less on Sunday, her one day off. She also feels energetic on dates or at parties, even during the workweek—no matter how tired she'd been during the day. This timing made me suspect that ambivalence on the job was provoking fatigue. A medical examination and a review of her psychological history showed no abnormality. Situational fatigue had to be considered.

At first she doubted that resistance to her job could show itself as fatigue. After all, the work wasn't hard, her salary was more than adequate, and she could come and go as she pleased. However, as we discussed her feelings about being a bookkeeper the fatigue connection made increasing sense. She was preoccupied, wondering if her father was type-casting her into a "woman's job."

I suggested that she had two choices. Change her job or change her attitude. As we talked, she recognized that her father felt insecure supervising the financial side of the business. He had given Jane the bookkeeping job because he needed someone he could trust to watch the finances. Jane also came to see that if she were to run the business one day, control over the financial side would be essential.

Our conversation also brought out a more subtle resistance. Jane was not really sure she wanted to run the company. She liked the idea of a family business and was thrilled that her sales work made a real contribution. However, she was not enthusiastic about supervising a three-shift assembly line, hiring and firing foremen, worrying about Hong Kong imports, and dealing with the union. That kind of responsibility could interfere with her other goals and priorities—marriage, family, skiing, reading, time to herself.

Jane realized that it wasn't necessary right now to make a decision about long-range goals. She could change her attitude about the bookkeeping job, however. She realized that her "job" was not just to do the books but to master them. Understanding this perspective told her that she was being offered the equivalent of a business-school course in fi-

Table 10.1: LIFE SITUATIONS INVENTORY

Potential Sources of Situational Fatigue	*Yes*	*No*	*Not Sure*
MARRIAGE/FAMILY RELATIONSHIPS			
Do you obtain enough emotional support?	_____	_____	_____
Have you a feeling of intimacy?	_____	_____	_____
Is there good communication among family members?	_____	_____	_____
Are you subject to excess criticism?	_____	_____	_____
Do you spend good time together with family?	_____	_____	_____
Are sexual relations satisfying?	_____	_____	_____
Are finances adequate?	_____	_____	_____
Is the family tone one of cooperation?	_____	_____	_____
Is arguing kept in proper proportion?	_____	_____	_____
Is there an atmosphere of respect?	_____	_____	_____
Are things well in your relationships with children, parents, and other relatives?	_____	_____	_____
WORK/SCHOOL			
Are you reasonably pleased with your financial position/school achievement?	_____	_____	_____
Do you find your work/school reasonably satisfying emotionally?	_____	_____	_____
Do you enjoy your social interaction with friends on the job/in school?	_____	_____	_____
Are you comfortable with the amount of responsibility and control you have in your work?	_____	_____	_____
Do your supervisors/teachers provide satisfactory supervision and support?	_____	_____	_____
Have you achieved proper recognition and appreciation for the work you have done?	_____	_____	_____
Are you optimistic about the future of your work/school?	_____	_____	_____
Is the amount of stress reasonable and capable of being handled?	_____	_____	_____
Are you comfortable with the number of hours you work?	_____	_____	_____
Is the physical setting of your work/school safe, clean, and congenial?	_____	_____	_____
Are you comfortable with the commuting you must do?	_____	_____	_____
PLAY			
Do you have enough free time?	_____	_____	_____
Do you have adequate time for recreation or hobbies?	_____	_____	_____
Do you have enough time for friends and acquaintances?	_____	_____	_____

Table 10.1: LIFE SITUATIONS INVENTORY (Cont.)

Potential Sources of Situational Fatigue	*Yes*	*No*	*Not Sure*
PLAY			
Do you have enough time for yourself?	_____	_____	_____
Are you satisfied with the uses you make of your free time?	_____	_____	_____
LIFE-STYLE			
Are you satisfied with your:			
physical shape	_____	_____	_____
eating and weight	_____	_____	_____
alcohol, tobacco, or drug use	_____	_____	_____
social status and prestige	_____	_____	_____
material possessions	_____	_____	_____
amount of rest and sleep	_____	_____	_____
freedom from time pressure	_____	_____	_____
degree of worry about the future	_____	_____	_____
LIVING QUARTERS			
Are your physical quarters comfortable?	_____	_____	_____
Are you able to handle the chores and repairs without undue distress?	_____	_____	_____
Is your neighborhood and are your neighbors a positive influence?	_____	_____	_____
Are you satisfied with regard to the physical environment (noise, pollution, etc.), pets, shopping, transportation?	_____	_____	_____
SPIRITUAL			
Do you have sense that your life has value, meaning, purpose, and fulfillment?	_____	_____	_____
Are you pleased with who you are as a person and with your system of values?	_____	_____	_____
Have you a satisfactory spiritual side to your life?	_____	_____	_____
Are you reasonably satisfied with the state of the world and its future?	_____	_____	_____
DISTRACTIONS AND ANNOYANCES			
Bureaucrats, bills, red lights, arguments—you name it!	_____	_____	_____
Your physical health and your family's	_____	_____	_____
Your mental health and your family's	_____	_____	_____

nancial management and the opportunity to take charge of a critical part of the business.

Jane began meeting regularly with the company accountant to understand cash flows, costs, and the bottom line: profit. She developed more interest in the books and she began to look forward to learning more about them each day. At the same time her energy increased.

Jane was tired because of boredom and dissatisfaction. Her job was not stressful in the usual sense. However, she was resisting it, and that resistance signaled itself as fatigue. At first she did not perceive the signal's meaning because she did not ask herself the key questions: "Why am I only tired at work—and why now?"

How to Recognize Your Situational Fatigue

Ask yourself if you are more than slightly dissatisfied with any aspect of your life. How long have you felt this way? Did anything change about the time you began to suffer from fatigue? Does your pattern of fatigue go up and down when you become more or less concerned about your dissatisfactions? Does it seem possible/plausible/likely that your fatigue is situational? If you improve this area of your life might your energy increase? Try it. Could you change your situation? Could you change your attitude?

Table 10.1 lists major areas of life that often generate situational fatigue. Run through the list rapidly. Check or circle those in which your satisfaction could be improved. Then go back and think about each one. Could it be the source of situational fatigue?

If you spot a potential problem area, think about it as you would a stress. Even if it's a small thing that should not be stressful, it might be a monumental drain on you. If so, review the guidelines in Chapter 6 for understanding stressful situations. Apply the stress management approaches to your situational fatigue.

CHAPTER

11

THE MIND/BODY INTERFACE

Conditioned Fatigue—An Unrecognized Ailment

Chronic fatigue from psychological causes sometimes strikes individuals who are the picture of mental health. Consider the experience of Fred Johnson, who developed leukemia at age thirty-two. Until then, he had everything going for him physically and mentally. But each dose of chemotherapy left him with nausea and profound fatigue. Now, three years since his last chemotherapy, Fred seems to be cured. He is nevertheless still plagued by attacks of nausea and fatigue—less disabling than during his chemotherapy, but still very distressing.

Attacks occur without apparent reason. However, Fred can count on them when he visits the doctor, thinks about chemotherapy, or is reminded of it by sounds, sights, or smells. He remembers, particularly, the perfume worn by the chemotherapy nurse. He becomes nervous when he smells anything like it. Between episodes Fred frequently worries about when his next "attack" will occur.

Is Fred's problem psychological? The psychiatrist says Fred does not seem to have a subconscious "need" to be "sick," as some people might, to escape distressing burdens or to elicit attention or care. Nor is his story unusual. A recent survey of cancer survivors showed that about 40 percent experienced symptoms resembling chemotherapy's side effects years after treatment had ceased.

As I thought about Fred's problem, I could not help remembering the great Russian physiologist Ivan Pavlov's training dogs to salivate at the sound of a bell. Dogs normally salivate when they see or smell meat—an automatic reflex. Pavlov took advantage of this by ringing a bell just when the meat would appear, forging an association between meat and the sound of the bell. Eventually Pavlov could ring the bell without giving meat and the dogs would still salivate. The innate reflex of salivation had been transferred to a very different stimulus, the sound of the bell. This process is known as conditioning.

Fred had a similar but less pleasant conditioning each time he had chemotherapy. Instead of a bell ringing, each chemotherapy triggered nausea and fatigue. Therefore I wondered: might Fred's toxic reaction to chemotherapy have been transferred to the sights, sounds, smells, and thoughts associated with his treatments? If so, what should be harmless stimuli would take on the power to trigger involuntary nausea and fatigue.

A fortunate characteristic of conditioned habits is that they eventually lose their power if the expected response doesn't occur. When Pavlov stopped providing meat, after a while the dogs would no longer salivate at the sound of the bell. I wondered if we might cure Fred's nausea/fatigue reaction by breaking the link between the reminders of his chemotherapy and his physical response.

Cancer specialists know that hypnosis can help prevent side effects such as nausea in persons actively on chemotherapy. We therefore asked Fred to take a short course of hypnosis which suggested that he would no longer react physically when he encountered reminders of his chemotherapy. He was to think, instead, of how effective the treatment had been in making him completely well. Within a few sessions, Fred's success was dramatic. Today, severe attacks almost never occur. As he gained control over his attacks his worry in anticipation of them also decreased.

Cindy Callas had a similar story, but in a very different context. She had been in excellent health until one year ago, when at twenty-four she developed a violent, week-long intestinal flu and high fever. Despite nausea and vomiting she forced fluids to prevent dehydration. She became nearly delirious and feared she might die. Even as she recovered she felt she was "falling apart."

Since then Cindy has not been herself. She is usually tired. Each day brings another distress: headaches one day, tingling hands another, diarrhea on a third—and sometimes all of them mixed together with dizziness, breathing difficulties, itching, and other odd symptoms. Food was particularly likely to provoke her, especially liquids.

Several thousand dollars of medical examination and testing had found nothing physically wrong. I raised the possibility that she might be suffering from a kind of conditioned reflex, learned involuntarily at the time of her intestinal illness. Had she, during those terrible days, come to associate the symptoms of her illness—headaches, diarrhea, and dizziness—with the liquids she had been forcing? She become so aware of even normal changes in her body every small twinge caused her body to say, in effect, "Oh no, here it comes again," triggering by reflex the biochemical changes that would produce debilitating tiredness and the other symptoms.

Cindy became extremely intent as we talked, her intuition heartily agreeing that this might be what had happened. She had a religious objection to hypnosis, so we offered her a technique known as guided visual imagery. We taught her to picture in her mind a scene of calm and tranquility, which would make her feel very relaxed. We asked her to invoke this image each time her symptoms even remotely threatened. She did this faithfully and within two weeks reported that she was symptom-free for the first time in a year.

Fred's and Cindy's cases are unusual because of their dramatic improvement and because the events triggering their problems were relatively easy to identify. Might others have acquired mysterious symptoms through more subtle conditioned reactions? The original source of conditioned responses can go back many years and be lost to memory. Even the specific triggers and associations might have become obscured as they in turn transferred their power to ordinary physiological processes and minor distresses that are routine in the body.

When I discussed this conditioning theory with an older relative, she told me a story she had been too embarrassed to share before. While in her twenties a dentist had given her too large a dose of an anesthetic containing adrenalin. Not surprisingly, she reacted with heart palpitations, sweating, and nervousness. While in this anxious state a trolley car rumbled by (this being in Brooklyn forty years ago). For the next two years each time she sat in the dentist's chair and heard the streetcar passing she would have a mini-panic attack. She knew these attacks were irrational, that she was not "allergic" to trolleys, yet it took two years for this involuntary reaction to fade.

Recent animal research suggests that conditioned learning of disease symptoms could be extremely important. For example, Dr. Robert Ader of the University of Rochester fed rats Cytoxan, a potent cancer chemotherapy agent. At the same time they drank water flavored with saccharin, a relatively benign artificial sweetener. Cytoxan normally reduces the count of certain immune cells in the blood. After a while, rats who had been exposed to saccharin and Cytoxan together developed immune cell reductions when they drank saccharin alone—just as if they had taken Cytoxan. Rats who had not been conditioned to associate Cytoxan with saccharin suffered no ill effects from saccharin. Scientists are debating whether the saccharin/Cytoxan conditioning affected the immune cells directly or indirectly by triggering a general stress reaction. Either way, this experiment shows that the power of a toxic substance is capable of being transferred to one that ordinarily does no harm.

In an equally fascinating experiment, researchers at the University of California induced allergy to egg in guinea pigs and then exposed the animals simultaneously to egg and to a particular pungent smell. Later, when presented with the smell by itself, these conditioned animals suffered an allergic reaction every bit as severe as that triggered by egg.

Neither Pavlov's dogs, Ader's rats, nor the allergic guinea pigs were "neurotic," "hysterical," or the victims of unconscious psychological conflict. Therefore, learning by conditioning is not a mental illness but a normal biological process that sometimes leads us astray. In a more optimistic perspective, conditioned learning can also be used to teach and condition our bodies when and how to relax. This can be done through relaxation exercises, biofeedback, hypnosis, or just plain "positive thinking."

Pavlovian conditioning as a cause of fatigue and other symptoms in humans has not been studied much, at least not outside Russia. I suspect it affects many people who are chronically ill from almost any disease. After all, when one feels bad much of the time there is ample opportunity to acquire accidental associations coincident to our symptoms. However, even if your symptoms are only partly the result of acquired conditioning, relief from even some of your triggers should be a blessing. I doubt that cases like Fred's and Cindy's are common—where conditioning is the main or only cause of the problem. On the other hand, they may not be rare. We won't know unless we make it a habit to look.

Anyone whose symptoms are not easily explained by physical disease, life stress, or (after evaluation by a psychiatrist) by internal emotional conflicts should consider that they might be at least partly caused by conditioning. This is especially likely if your symptoms had a well-defined onset over a few months or less following a period of intense physical or emotional upset. If special situations, thoughts, foods, sights, or smells seem to affect you, consider if they are reminiscent of the circumstances in which this illness began or other situations when you were not well.

Finally, recognize that the ability to acquire conditioned responses does not imply any weakness of mind. To the contrary, all cases I have identified have been among individuals of above-average intelligence. Most have exceptionally powerful minds when it comes to creative or imaginative tasks.

Treatment. For a few of my patients, just gaining insight about how conditioning works and how it might affect their fatigue has been enough to disarm their conditioned responses. Others take six to ten sessions of training in visual imagery, self-hypnosis, stress management, and relaxation techniques designed to replace negative conditioning cues with positive, helpful responses. About 60 percent of those for whom conditioned problems seem likely improve as a result of this program. Most are not cured, but their symptoms occur less often and less intensely. In general, we have observed that physical stress such as viral infections, dietary indiscretion, and lack of sleep tend to worsen "conditioned" symptoms, as does any form of emotional trauma. Sensible self-care and personal tranquility foster improvement.

If the message of this section might apply to you, discuss it with your physician or a psychologist, preferably one with some understanding of such behavioral methods as hypnosis, guided visual imagery, or relaxation techniques. A few physicians and quite a few psychologists have skills in these areas. Some health professionals who have an interest in behavioral medicine may not be technically skilled in actually applying the techniques. In these cases noncertified workers such as a hypnotechnician can be helpful. Such people should work under the close guidance of a physician or psychologist. It is not proper for a hypnotechnician or other nonprofessional to treat you medically or psychologically without formal supervision.

Fatigue That Might Be "All in the Mind"

The psychiatrists' official *Diagnostic and Statistical Manual* describes a group of people with many physical symptoms for which no physical cause can be found. They *assume* this syndrome is purely psychiatric in origin, although the truth of this assumption has not been proved scientifically. Because these conditions mimic physical illness they are called somatoform disorders (*soma* in Greek means "body"). Many if not most of the people in this group are frequently tired.

Persons who fit the psychiatrist's definition of having somatoform disorders are well represented among those who complain year after year about chronic fatigue and many other symptoms.

Among the somatoform disorders, the most common type is known as a somatization disorder. Its victims are almost always female and their complaints almost always begin before age thirty. Their complaints have been medical and they have seen many doctors, rarely obtaining more than temporary relief. Individuals who suffer from extensive complaints for years without relief are often and understandably angry, frustrated, and skeptical of conventional medicine and psychiatry. They are not faking symptoms and do feel discomfort. Their physicians and psychiatrists may be equally exasperated and are often reluctant to treat them.

The characteristic symptoms of somatization disorder are listed in Table 11.1.

Not surprisingly, many individuals who show the characteristics of somatization disorder eventually seek help from nonphysicians or from unorthodox approaches including chiropractic, clinical ecology, megavitamins, acupuncture, hypoglycemia, candida yeast treatment, and the like. Many claim to benefit from these treatments. However, most skeptical physicians argue that if these treatments "work" it is because unorthodox practitioners give a name to the illness that puts the blame

Table 11.1: THE PSYCHIATRIC DEFINITION OF SOMATIZATION DISORDER

There is a feeling of unusual susceptibility to illness for most of one's life.

Over the years one has sought care for at least 14 of the following 37 symptoms or problems to the point of consulting a doctor, taking medicines, or altering one's lifestyle:

- Neurological-type symptoms: difficulty swallowing, loss of voice, deafness, double vision, blurred vision, blindness, fainting, memory loss, seizures or convulsions, trouble walking, paralysis or muscle weakness, urinary retention or difficulty urinating.
- Gastrointestinal symptoms: abdominal pain, nausea, vomiting spells (other than during pregnancy), bloating (gassy), intolerance to a variety of foods, diarrhea.
- Female reproductive symptoms: unusually painful menstruation, menstrual irregularity, excessive bleeding, severe vomiting throughout pregnancy.
- Psychosexual symptoms: sexual indifference, lack of pleasure or pain during intercourse.
- Pain: pain in back, joints, extremities or genital area, pain on urination, other pain (except for headache).
- Cardiopulmonary symptoms: shortness of breath, palpitations, chest pain, dizziness.

Adapted from *The Diagnostic and Statistical Manual,* vol. 3, American Psychiatric Association, 1980.

outside the patient, take advantage of the patient's desire to improve (the placebo effect), and provide more sympathetic support than do orthodox physicians. If this explanation is correct, something important is missing from mainstream medicine. However, most unorthodox practitioners believe that they are doing more than providing sympathy. Unfortunately, there have been few credible studies of the effects of unorthodox treatments on somatization disorder—or, for that matter, on almost anything else.

To be fair, psychiatrists don't actually claim to understand why somatization disorder occurs. Nor is classical psychiatry effective at treating it. This combination of no cause and no treatment is a sure prescription for frustration and distrust.

Probably some victims really have physical disorders. For example, if the diagnosis of chronic Epstein-Barr virus syndrome proves valid, it will provide physical explanation for the symptoms of one group of individuals who would otherwise be diagnosed as having somatization disorder. Others may have subtle disorders of the endocrine glands, porphyria (a rare metabolic disorder), multiple sclerosis, systemic lupus erythematosus (an autoimmune disorder), or an odd seizure disorder. Others may have variants of treatable psychiatric conditions such as panic anxiety, depression, or schizophrenia.

Perhaps somatization problems are mainly psychiatric. If so, why are almost all victims young women? Why do so many also show subtle abnormalities of endocrine function? Are these endocrine findings the effect of the disease or a key to its hidden physical basis? Many of the somatization patients we encounter are exquisitely sensitive to the side effects of medicine. Is this "psychological" or does it reflect a difference in their metabolic processing of drugs and other chemicals?

If your symptoms fit the pattern of somatization disorder, obtain a psychiatric evaluation (but be sure your doctor has also looked for physical causes). If psychotherapy is suggested, ask frankly about the likelihood that you will benefit. Ideally, you should feel there are important psychological issues in your life worth working on even if your psychotherapy did not help your fatigue and other bodily symptoms.

Neither relaxation approaches such as yoga, meditation, or biofeedback nor "mind-training" approaches such as guided visual imagery and self-hypnosis will cure somatization disorder, although these treatments sometimes reduce the severity of symptoms.

Hypochondriasis is a different type of somatoform disorder. The hypochondriac is not so much ill or feeling bad as worried. Every little twinge is interpreted as the possible sign of a dread disease such as cancer, heart disease, or AIDS. This unrealistic fear, which affects men and women equally, usually sets in before middle age. These fears persist despite medical evaluation finding no disease. Hypochondriacal worrying, as might be expected, can lead to fatigue as well as to anxiety and depression. Because of the hypochondriac's "'wolf'-crying" history, when physical illness does occur it can easily be missed. Psychiatric treatment can be helpful in understanding the underlying psychological basis for the hypochondriac's fears and in reducing them.

Hysterical or conversion disorder should not be confused with either hypochondriasis or somatization disorder. It is relatively rare and is not a common cause of chronic fatigue. However, conversion disorder is the best known of the somatoform disorders because Freud wrote about it and suffered from it himself. In this century wartime "shell shock" is the best-known example.

Hysterical conversion of mental anguish into physical symptoms is what we often have in mind when we say "It's all in your head." Unbearable trauma, physical or psychological, can cause the mind, in effect, to partly shut down. The result is odd symptoms such as paralysis, inability to talk, blindness, or numbness or pain that anatomy cannot explain. In a sense the mind changes physical reality to protect itself from emotional pain. Psychiatric treatment is often effective, with hypnosis being a valuable tool. Conversion hysteria might be related in some ways to another disorder that can cause chronic fatigue, post-traumatic stress disorder, discussed briefly in Chapter 6.

PART 3

MEDICINES AND DRUGS THAT MAKE YOU TIRED

CHAPTER

12

PRESCRIPTION AND NONPRESCRIPTION MEDICINES, ALCOHOL, AND DRUGS OF ABUSE

Follow one cardinal rule in trying to understand baffling symptoms: suspect any medicine a person is taking. Fatigue is one of the most common side effects of medicines. Since Americans fill two billion prescriptions each year and 75 million of us take one or more medicines each week, medication-induced fatigue is a major national problem. Side effects of medicine can be difficult to recognize because, when they develop gradually, you may not be aware of their effect until after you stop taking the drug. Some medicines are very likely to cause fatigue: antihistamine cold medicines, sleeping pills, antiulcer drugs, many high blood pressure medicines. Some cause tiredness less often or only in special circumstances: birth control pills, diuretics, diet aids, and anti-inflammatory pain medicines.

Be especially suspicious of any medicine you began taking within a few months of first noticing fatigue. However, question *every* drug—even those that you started long before or long after your problem began.

Consider the situation of Tim Jones, a thirty-five-year-old school guidance counselor. Two years ago, immediately following his divorce, he became tired and depressed. His family physician placed him on antidepressant medicines and referred him for counseling. His depression improved but his tiredness continued. His doctor thought this meant he was still depressed. He increased the dose of the antidepressant medicine. However, Tim became more fatigued . . . and more frustrated. One day he threw his pills away; within a week his fatigue had vanished.

Tim Jones' depression had ended long ago. It was the antidepressant medicine that still kept him tired.

Mrs. J.P., a fifty-year-old-housewife, had been tired and weak for about six months. About two months later she developed heart palpitations.

She had been taking a diuretic pill for high blood pressure for about six years. Although her diuretic medicine can deplete potassium, it had not been rechecked for several years. In fact, her blood-potassium level turned out to be low. A liquid potassium supplement restored it to normal. To her delight, fatigue and palpitations both disappeared.

M.L., fourteen years old, took a medicine called theophylline. His doctor had explained that theophylline, a close cousin of caffeine, might make him nervous. This was not a problem, but after a month the boy began to have difficulty keeping awake in school. He couldn't sleep well at night, another side effect of theophylline. His doctor switched him to Intal, a nonstimulating antiasthma drug. M.L. slept well again and his daytime fatigue disappeared.

Medicines

These cases illustrate the importance of reviewing all medicines with your doctor. Keep this specific question in mind: Is it possible that my medicine is contributing to my fatigue? For at least half the most commonly taken medicines the answer could be yes. However, *you cannot simply drop a medicine that you suspect may be causing fatigue. That could be extremely dangerous.* Decide with your doctor whether you can afford a medicine-free holiday or whether a less-tiring medicine might serve as a substitute.

The "official" information sheet for a typical drug may list fifty or more potential side effects, often including fatigue. Your doctor cannot explain them all to you when he or she prescribes a drug. You must therefore inform your physician if you develop new symptoms. You should also do "homework" on the medicines you are taking.

The following pages discuss the fatigue-inducing potential of each of the main types of prescription and over-the-counter or nonprescription drugs. Appendix 6 contains a specific evaluation of the fatigue potential for each of the 150 most frequently prescribed medicines. Finally, we will describe references from which you can learn about your medicines in more detail.

Antibiotics. These kill bacteria, fungi, or parasites. Fatigue is not a usual side effect.

Antidepressant medicines. The most popular type, the tricyclic antidepressants, routinely cause fatigue and sometimes mental cloudiness.

Examples: Adapin, Aventyl, Elavil, Imipramine, Ludiomil, Sinequan, Tofranil. Desyrel is a relatively new antidepressant that is much like the tricylics.

The other main type of antidepressant is called a MAO (monoamine oxidase) inhibitor. It has much less potential for fatigue, although it has its own types of other side effects. Examples: Marplan, Nardil.

Antihistamines. This class of drugs is most often used to relieve the nasal symptoms of colds or allergies. These substances also suppress hives, and a few help combat dizziness and motion sickness. All but one of the commercially available antihistamine medicines typically cause fatigue. The common practice of packaging antihistamines in combination with stimulating decongestant drugs often reduces fatigue as a side effect. Seldane (terfenadine) is available as a nonsedating antihistamine. Others should be on the market within a year or two.

Examples: Atarax, Benadryl, Brompheniramine, Chlor-trimeton, Dimetane, Dimetapp, Phenergan, Tavist, Vistaril.

Asthma medicines. Most (but not all) asthma medicines are stimulants. Typical side effects include nervousness, anxiety, and difficulty sleeping. Fatigue can result indirectly from overstimulation or from poor-quality sleep. The inhaled versions of these medicines provoke less-intense side effects than those taken by mouth.

Examples: Alupent, Brethine, Elixophyllin, Metaprel, Proventil, Slo-Phyllin, Theo-dur, theophylline, Ventolin.

Beta blockers. These medications block the effect of the hormone adrenalin and are useful in treating angina heart disease, high blood pressure, heartbeat irregularities, migraine headache, and even stage fright. Certain brands claim less fatigue potential, but I consider all beta blockers to have potential for causing fatigue, weakness, and dizziness or depression.

Examples: Corgard, Inderal, Lopressor, Normodyne, Tenormin, Trandate, Visken.

Calcium channel blockers. A recent development, these drugs are useful in most of the same conditions for which we use beta blockers. Fatigue-related complaints occur in a small but significant minority of patients.

Examples: Calan, Cardizem, Isoptin, Procardia.

Cold/allergy/cough medicines. Usually these contain one or more of the following: antihistamines, which often cause fatigue; decongestants, which can cause overstimulation; and cough suppressants (usually natural or synthetic codeine), which can cause fatigue. Their sedating and stimulating side effects often balance—but not always.

Diet medicines. There are three main types: fiber or bulking agents, which are no problem; low-calorie powder or pudding food substitutes; and appetite suppressants. Low-calorie food substitutes taken without adequate food can cause metabolic imbalances, fatigue, and more dangerous complications. Appetite suppressants usually contain potent stimulants that can cause nervousness and fatigue. Stopping them can lead to withdrawal tiredness and depression.

Examples: Dexatrim, Dexedrine, Phentermine, Pondimin, Preludin, Sanorex, Trimtabs.

Diuretics. Important medicines for high blood pressure, heart failure, and certain liver and kidney diseases, diuretics promote increased urination. They do not cause fatigue directly but can do so indirectly if they promote dehydration or too low a blood pressure. Many, but not all, deplete the body of potassium and magnesium, which can bring on fatigue.

Examples: Aladactazide, Bumex, Dyazide, Esidrix, Hydrodiuril (hydrochlorthiazide), Lasix (furosemide), Moduretic, Zaroxolyn.

Gastrointestinal drugs. There are an immense number of gastrointestinal symptoms and an immense number of drugs for each. Except for antacids and most laxatives, almost all can cause fatigue, dizziness, or related symptoms.

For example: antiulcer drugs (Tagamet, Zantac); antispasm drugs (Bentyl, Donnatal, Librax, Pro-Banthine); gastrointestinal stimulants (Reglan); antidiarrhea medicines (Imodium, Lomotil).

Heart medicines. Digitalis type heart medicine causes few side effects when the dose is right. However, its margin of safety is narrow. Too much can result in apathy, weakness, fatigue, and depression. Low blood-potassium levels due to diuretics as well as small changes in the efficiency of the kidney can cause serious digitalis complications.

Examples: digoxin, Lanoxin, digitalis.

Nitroglycerin products, the most common treatment for angina chest pain, do not cause fatigue directly. However, they can cause low blood pressure, which in turn can cause fatigue.

Examples: Isordil, Nitro-Bid, nitroglycerin, Nitrostat, Sorbitrate.

Various drugs used to correct or prevent irregular heart rhythm can produce fatigue in some individuals.

Examples: Quinaglute, quinidine, Pronestyl, Norpace, beta blockers, calcium channel blockers.

High blood pressure medicines. Many, but not all, have substantial potential for causing fatigue. Beta blockers, calcium channel blockers, and diuretics are discussed separately above. High blood pressure medicines that often cause fatigue include Aldomet, Catapres, Ismelin, Minpress, and Reserpine.

Any high blood pressure treatment can cause fatigue if too low a blood pressure results.

Hormones. The most frequently taken are birth control pills. These can produce many side effects, including depression and fatigue. Too high a dose of thyroid hormone can cause fatigue through overstimulation. Adrenal steroids such as prednisone and medrol have many side effects, fatigue and mood changes among them.

Pain medicines. There are three main kinds: anti-inflammatory medicines, which help fever and pain; narcotic pain medicines; and others. Anti-inflammatory pain medicines cause fatigue in a significant minority of people as well as dizziness and mental sluggishness.

Examples: Aspirin in all its many brand names, and also Advil, Anaprox, Feldene, Indocin, Motrin, Nalfon, Nuprin, phenylbutazone, Ponstel, Rufen, Tolectin.

Narcotic pain medicines all have potential for sedation, fatigue, and physical or psychological dependence. Examples: Codeine, Darvon, Demerol, Morphine, Percodan, Talwin.

Most other pain medicines, such as acetaminophen (Tylenol), do not have fatigue as a major side effect.

Sleeping medicines. Sleeping medicines are supposed to make you tired. However, for many, the sedation lasts into the next day. This morning-after effect depends on how fast your metabolism works to dispose of the drug. Halcion has the shortest length of action and is least likely to cause daytime sedation.

Examples: Dalmane, Halcion, Restoril, Seconal.

Tranquilizers. The so-called minor tranquilizers are used for moderately intense anxiety, muscle relaxation, and occasionally as sleeping pills. Sedation and fatigue are common.

Examples: Ativan, Centrax, Librium, Miltown, Valium.

Major tranquilizers treat extreme anxiety and also major psychiatric problems such as schizophrenia. Properly used, they are invaluable, but sedation and mental clouding are common reactions.

Examples: Haldol, Mellaril, Serantil, Thorazine.

Compazine, a potent antinausea drug, is related to the major tranquilizers. It also tends to cause fatigue.

A new type of tranquilizer, Bus-Par, does not sedate but does sometimes cause overstimulation.

Appendix 6 lists the most commonly used prescription drugs. The same medicines can go by several names. Every drug has a chemical or generic name. Many also have one or more trademark or brand names that drug companies use in their advertising.

The first table in the appendix gives the 150 most popular prescription drugs and their potential for fatigue. I have excluded antibiotics and creams, since these rarely cause fatigue. Listings are usually by brand names unless the generic name is also frequently used in writing prescriptions.

If your prescription drug is not in the alphabetical listing of Appendix Table 1, look for it in Table 2, which gives the most popular generic names and their brand-name equivalents. You can then find the brand name in Table 1.

If your medicine is not on either table or if you wish to learn more about it, check any of the following references. Of course, take specific questions directly to your physician or pharmacist.

Drug References

The *PDR* or *Physician's Desk Reference* (Medical Economics Company, Oradell, NJ) is the most widely used. It describes almost every prescription drug. A companion volume discusses nonprescription drugs. You can find them in almost every library and in many bookstores.

The *PDR* has two main problems for general readers: it is written for doctors and it is a legal document. Its language is technical; even the table of contents is a challenge. Legally, every possible side effect gets listed. The *PDR* can be extremely useful, but it offers great potential for confusion.

The Package Insert. Most prescription drugs come to the pharmacist with a detailed leaflet describing the drug. Your pharmacist should give you a copy if you ask for it. Usually the package insert is identical to the drug's description in the *PDR.*

Advice for the Patient (Rockville, Md.: United States Pharmacopeia Convention, Inc.)
Much better for patients than the *PDR.* It distinguishes common reactions from rare ones and is written clearly. The index is logical.

The Essential Guide to Prescription Drugs by Dr. James Long. (New York: Harper & Row)
Very good and very comprehensive. Written by a thinking person rather than by a computer or a potential defense attorney.

The Pill Book by Dr. Harold Silverman. (New York: Bantam Books)
Smaller and more selective than Dr. Long's book, but also a fine resource.

The People's Pharmacy series by Joe Graedon. (New York: St.Martin's Press)
Partly reference books and partly personal opinion essays. Intelligent and fun to read.

Alcohol and Drugs of Abuse

If most of us have too much to drink, we can't think clearly that day and may sleep poorly that night. We understand that too much alcohol is the reason we feel bad. However, fatigue due to alcohol is actually much more common than most of us imagine.

People who drink every day get accustomed to alcohol's effects. Many proclaim "It doesn't affect me," not recognizing the many ways that alcohol drains our minds and our bodies. You don't have to be an alcoholic to fall into this trap.

Most of us can drink moderately with no major harm. However, long before you become ill, alcohol can contribute to your fatigue. Many people sleep less deeply if they drink before bedtime. Alcohol can depress the pumping power of the heart. Its effects on the kidneys are well known. It can reduce resistance to infection as well as to stress. The moral is that if you drink even a little almost every day, you should find out if alcohol is affecting you. How you feel after several weeks away from all alcohol should tell you the answer. Of course, millions of

Americans have a problem that goes beyond feeling tired. If you feel genuinely deprived when you cannot drink, or "need" a drink to relax or feel good, you'd best look again. Whether or not you are actually addicted to alcohol—suffer anxiety, irritability, hallucinations, or seizures on its withdrawal—the potential for alcoholism is probably present.

Alcohol as a problem drug is more common than most people realize. Authorities estimate that between 5 percent and 10 percent of our adult population might be affected to a degree. Perhaps 20 percent of medical admissions to a community hospital are alcohol-related, directly or indirectly. However, except for the case of the obvious alcoholic, most people (including physicians!) usually fail to recognize the pattern of alcohol abuse.

This oversight can be tragic. Alcohol has been linked to about half of all automobile accidents, half of all murders, a quarter of suicides, and about 40 percent of problems brought to family court. The economic loss is estimated at over $100 billion each year.

People who drink too often, too intensely, or for the wrong reasons often deny there is a problem long after friends or family suspect it. Partly this is from shame or a fear of being found out. However, it is also from pride, a false pride perhaps, that you are strong enough to handle alcohol, that it will not get the best of you. . . .

Suspect that you may be abusing alcohol if you have ever felt you should cut down on your drinking, if people annoyed you by criticizing your drinking, if you have ever felt bad or guilty about drinking, or if you have ever had a drink first thing in the morning to steady your nerves or get rid of a hangover.

You might drink simply because you enjoy it, or as a kind of self-medication to help you relax or forget your problems. However, you can easily become trapped in a vicious cycle that leads to a chemical dependency.

If you drink regularly, part of the evaluation of your fatigue should be a several-week holiday away from all alcohol. If that thought seems upsetting, offensive, or ridiculous ask if this might itself be a sign that something is wrong. One caution, though, if you become nervous or jittery when you omit or postpone an accustomed drink, is that your body may already be addicted. In that case, talk to your physician before doing anything. Sudden withdrawal from alcohol can cause serious problems.

Alcohol is our most pervasive problem drug. We also face others.

The National Institute of Drug Abuse estimates that there may be two million cocaine addicts and that half of Americans aged twenty-five to thirty have sampled cocaine. Cocaine is like caffeine multiplied a million times—it boosts you meteorically and drops you absolutely, exhausting your nervous system. This cause of fatigue should be obvious despite the immense power of self-delusion.

Marijuana smokers recognize pot's acute powers of sedation but may not realize that this drug remains in the body for many days after it is taken. If you take marijuana two or three times a week, don't be surprised if you are tired all the time.

Tobacco is another route to mild stimulation followed by a let-down that calls for yet another pick-me-up—the next cigarette or coffee or both. This stress-fatigue seesaw can wear you out by itself. Tobacco also constricts blood vessels, so the heart must pump harder; compromises the respiratory system, demanding more effort to breathe; and pushes the entire metabolism into high gear. Ex-smokers sometimes marvel at how alive they feel once they kick their habit. (They should be overjoyed, as well, by how much longer they will be alive!)

The list of abusable drugs is long and includes prescription drugs such as diet pills and sleeping pills as well as such illegal drugs as heroin and LSD. Many users think they can handle them. Chronic fatigue can be the first indicator that their judgment was poor.

PART 4

PHYSICAL ENVIRONMENT AND FATIGUE

CHAPTER

13

HOME, WORKPLACE, AND OUTDOORS

You don't have to be a meteorologist to know that the physical environment affects how you feel, but it is amazing how often this is overlooked when evaluating the causes of chronic fatigue. This chapter is about the physical environment: the light we see by, the chemicals in our air and food, the noise of our surroundings, its electrical and magnetic charges, and the physical hazards of the office and home.

Lighting

SUNLIGHT AND ENERGY

Sandra M, a New Yorker, has fatigue and depression every winter. January vacations in Florida restore her good mood. During her doldrums she can't fall asleep before 1:00 A.M. but she often oversleeps in the morning.

Her doctor has found a way to return her sleep to normal, increase her energy, and relieve her depression. All this results when she merely exposes herself each morning to special bright lights designed to imitate sunlight.

Jason D is also tired and depressed. In contrast to Sandra, he' collapses each night before 10:00 P.M. but awakes feeling tired at 4:30 A.M.. His fatigue lack's Sandra's seasonal pattern, but his symptoms are also relieved by bright lights. Jason's lights, however, go on in the evening.

Light may be critical to how we feel. Everyone "knows" that short winter days and dark, somber colors tend to dampen one's mood. However, until recently most physicians classed these beliefs with folk myths and old wives' tales.

In the early 1970s John Ott, a former Disney photographer, wrote a controversial book suggesting that ordinary indoor light lacks key elements of natural sunlight that are important for maintaining energy and good health.

In the mid-1970s scientists at Cornell University confirmed part of Ott's theory. "Full-spectrum" lights, designed to simulate sunlight, seemed better than ordinary indoor light in preventing psychological fatigue. By 1980 researchers at the National Institutes of Health had identified a new disease, Seasonal Affective Disorder (SAD). Its victims tend to become depressed each winter and recover each spring. SAD may result from too little bright sunlight, which triggers biochemical abnormalities in the brain of especially sensitive individuals. Very bright full-spectrum light sometimes relieves this disorder within a matter of days.

Seasonal Affective Disorder might be just the tip of an iceberg of mood and energy problems related to light. Our knowledge is too primitive to know with certainty. If you become fatigued or depressed when the days grow short, it makes sense to see if a Southern vacation helps. Or make a habit of getting outside for an hour early each sunny morning and again at midday. (Be sure to go to sleep earlier to make up for sleep lost in the morning.)

Setting up full-spectrum lights in your home might be an option for the future, but the very bright lights researchers use to treat SAD are not presently sold in stores. As important, we are just learning to use light properly. There might even be side effects in certain individuals, so recommendations for self-treatment cannot yet be given.

FLUORESCENT LIGHT

R.T. is a prominent allergist. While inspecting slides mounted on a fluorescent-light viewing box he had to rest every few minutes. Fluorescent lights, he said, cause him fatigue. He avoids them whenever possible.

A fair number of people complain that fluorescent lights make them tired, spacy, nauseous, or headachy—at least after long exposure. They may become uncomfortable in supermarkets, department stores, or modern offices whose lighting can be a hidden cause of fatigue.

There are several theories why fluorescent light can be a problem. Its brightness can create an uncomfortable glare. This causes eye strain, which can cause fatigue. Fluorescent lights also flicker, somewhat like the strobe lights at a disco. This is wearying to some and may also contribute to fatigue. Extreme flickering (not that of standard fluorescent lights) can actually provoke epileptic seizures. Flickering possibly has a direct effect on the brain.

Fluorescent light emits ultraviolet radiation, high doses of which can cause skin cancer as well as fatigue. However, most experts doubt the amount of radiation in fluorescent light can be harmful. White plastic shields on the lights reduce ultraviolet exposure while decreasing glare. Another problem is the harsh and slightly greenish color created by the standard "cool white" fluorescent bulb. "Warmer" bulbs are available, including those which reasonably mimic natural sunlight.

If you are uncomfortable with fluorescent illumination and have a choice, substitute incandescent light or, better still, natural sunlight.

How much light? Both too much and too little light cause fatigue, eyestrain, headache, and other problems. The amount of light needed differs with the task. Reading a smudged photocopy requires twice as much light as reading a fine copy. Work on a computer screen (video display terminal) should be done in relatively low light, or glare will be a problem. Older individuals tend to require more light for the same task than young people. The aging eye is also more sensitive to glare.

Standard lighting in most offices inevitably provides too much light for some and too little for others. Ideally, each worker should be able to control his own light intensity.

Color and Mood. There is a large popular psychological literature about the effect of color on mood. Red is said to increase tension (seeing red) and raise blood pressure. Blue is said to do the reverse (feeling blue). Scientific studies on these effects have had inconsistent results. However, color does seem to influence some people.

Researchers at the University of Wales have confirmed previous findings that long-wavelength colors (red, orange, and yellow) tend to induce feelings of high arousal while short-wavelength colors (blue, indigo, and violet) induced low arousal. At different times, high arousal was experienced differently— sometimes as pleasant excitement, at other times as disturbing anxiety. Low arousal was experienced as pleasant relaxation at some times and as boredom at others. As an individual's preference for high versus low arousal changes throughout the day, his or her color preference may also change.

There may be other effects of color on mood. Some people believe they are warmer in a red room and cooler in a blue room. Some see a red wall as being closer and a blue one as farther away. Gamblers may tend toward riskier bets when playing under red lights than under blue lights. Submariners find low-level white light pleasanter than either blue or red.

There may be an inherent biological response to colors. However, most color-mood associations are probably learned by experience as conditioned reactions, or as part of one's culture. If particular colors tend to lift your mood or others depress it, respect those impressions. Surround yourself, if you can, with walls, rugs, and decorations that enhance your sense of well-being.

Chemicals in Our Environment

I once made a literal house call—for a house! The patient was a sick building. It was a new energy-efficient office without a single window that could be opened. Many occupants had complained of fatigue, headache, nasal stuffiness, and/or dizziness. The owners were frantic that this "mass hysteria" might jeopardize their multimillion-dollar investment.

The energy crisis of the 1970s led to a generation of well-insulated but poorly ventilated buildings. Since then complaints linking fatigue, headache, and respiratory symptoms to indoor air quality have multiplied. Yet no one is sure why "tight" buildings provoke symptoms. In a few cases there has been clear-cut indoor air pollution: tobacco smoke, rug shampoo, industrial chemicals, formaldehyde vapors, photocopy-machine chemicals. However, the majority of "sick buildings" show only a modest, across-the-board increase of common chemicals and pollutants, with no one element reaching levels that are considered toxic.

Most authorities feel that the common denominator is poor ventilation. Increasing fresh air usually solves the problem.

If your workplace is tightly sealed, and if you and many co-workers suffer from fatigue, headaches, and nasal symptoms, consider that indoor air pollution and inadequate ventilation might be the problem. Indoor air pollution can also occur at home, as you will see in a later section.

"Allergies" to chemicals. "Sick buildings" normally affect a large proportion of occupants, but Ed T was the only person in his laboratory who became sick.

Ed was a chemist who had become increasingly sensitive to chemicals he worked with. Within minutes after exposure he'd develop eye irritation, sinus-area headaches, a stuffy nose, profound fatigue, and difficulty concentrating. Soon his symptoms began appearing after exposures to everyday substances such as auto fumes, synthetic fabrics, and scented toilet tissue.

Ed had become what the clinical ecologists call a universal reactor—sensitive to everything. A dedicated worker, Ed struggled on. He even wore a respirator mask to his laboratory. His employers, alarmed, sent him to an occupational health physician, two psychiatrists, and an allergist. None could explain Ed's devastating illness.

No one knows why rare individuals develop overwhelming reactions to small doses of chemicals that cause no problems for others. One theory is that this is a kind of allergy. Chemical allergies do happen. There are a few definite cases of allergy to formaldehyde, carbonless carbon paper, photocopy-machine fumes, and certain industrial chemicals. However, unlike Ed, these victims usually react to only one or two chemicals. Another theory is that this is all psychological, a civilian version of shell-shock hysteria. Others argue that chemicals can irritate nerve endings or block metabolic function. These might generate nerve impulses or biochemical reactions that disrupt the brain or other vital organs.

Ed's sensitivity is extreme and unusual; however, many individuals suffer from chemical or smell sensitivity to a milder degree. Common offenders include tobacco smoke, perfume, household cleaners, detergents, and newsprint. Individuals with asthma or migraine headaches and pregnant women are particularly vulnerable. In addition to fatigue, typical symptoms include headache, nausea, breathlessness, nervousness, upset stomach.

I first treated Ed with sinus-headache medicines. These helped only a little. His symptoms progressed and Ed was placed on disability. He could avoid severe symptoms when secluded at home. However, trips to the store were sure to cause problems. Psychotherapy helped Ed fight his frustration, but did not affect his "allergies."

HYPNOSIS: A SURPRISING REMEDY

A year later, after I'd became interested in medical hypnosis, I asked Ed to learn self-hypnosis and condition himself not to react to a particular chemical. He tried this before exposing himself to the chemical. He reacted, but less intensely and for a shorter period than usual. The second time his reaction was less and the third time he did not react at all.

During the next four months Ed reversed about 70 percent of his chemical sensitivities. He was still limited in his activities, but very much improved. Then a peculiar series of events occurred.

Ed's father suffered a heart attack and was in unstable condition. Immediately, Ed began reacting to all the excitants that had bothered him at his worst—including such bizarre triggers as turning on the microwave oven. Then his father recovered, and Ed regained all his lost ground within a matter of days.

Ed's reactions to chemicals were real and disabling. Psychotherapy alone had little impact. Nevertheless, mental processes did have a profound effect, as demonstrated by the influence of stress and hypnosis. I don't know how much of Ed's problem is physical and how much is mental. Indeed, such distinctions may not be appropriate, since the two are inextricably intertwined. What is clear is that there are individual's who share Ed's vulnerability so that exposure to ordinary chemicals can trigger fatigue. This type of problem is also discussed in Chapter 11.

Chemical toxins. We are immersed in chemicals from the moment of conception. Most chemicals we encounter were introduced to the environment within recent memory, so we know little about potential long-term hazards. Many are immediately toxic if we are exposed to high doses. Cancer and birth defects may result later. The unanswered question is whether chronic low-dose exposures, which are extremely common, make us vulnerable to health problems, including fatigue. Concern is warranted, judging from what we already know from our unintended "experiments."

In Michigan during the 1970s, a fire retardant called PBB was accidentally mixed into cattle and chicken feed. Thousands of dairy cattle and more than a million chickens were destroyed, but only after thousands of Michigan farmers and their customers had eaten contaminated dairy or poultry products. This scandal received wide publicity and Michigan physicians recorded thousands of health complaints that people feared were related to eating food containing PBB. Were their symptoms coincidence? Were they from stress, anger, or fear induced by publicity and economic hardship? Or were they due to PBB?

Researchers from New York's Mount Sinai Hospital studied many Michigan farmers and their customers. They found PBB in their blood three years after the exposure. Wisconsin farmers, who were not exposed, showed no PBB. The Michigan residents also had an unusually high frequency of "stresslike" health complaints including fatigue, backache, numbness, tingling, weakness, sleepiness, nervousness, blurred vision, headache, and nausea. They also had subtle defects in the function of their immune cells. Again, Wisconsin farmers did not.

Were these changes in the immune system the direct result of the PBB? Or were they caused by continuing emotional stress and fear? For the time being, no one can say for sure. The issue is important to our health and to that of our children.

Even disregarding vast disasters such as that at Bhopal, India (where thousands died from uncontrolled industrial vapors), hundreds of major toxic chemical spills occur each year. Industrial waste sites leak in New Jersey. Missouri roads are coated with cancer-causing Dioxin. In Scotland, downwind from a chemical factory hundreds of livestock herds are decimated. More than sixty European wines are contaminated with antifreeze.

Less spectacular spills are now commonplace. Almost every American eating a "normal" diet has pesticides measurable in the blood. Even fish from the deep ocean accumulate the carcinogen PCB. It is theoretically plausible that our chemical burden reduces the efficiency of our body, increasing our vulnerability to fatigue and to more serious problems. Whether this actually occurs and whether it is common or rare are critical questions that have not been given the attention they deserve.

If you have a specific concern about an environmental chemical, your best resource is your state environmental protection agency or department of health. There are very few nongovernment physicians trained in environmental medicine. However, if you know which chemicals you are looking for, measuring their presence in your body or environment can be accomplished.

Noise stress. Noise is a psychological and a physical stressor. It can make you tired or give you a headache. Acutely, noise can raise your blood pressure, stress your adrenal glands, and affect your immune system. I am not talking about the extreme noises that can damage your hearing, such as industrial machinery or disco music. Much lower levels like the whir of a food blender or Manhattan street traffic can be a problem. One classic study found significant symptoms of stress in people affected by the noise of a nearby airport. Even lower levels such as the air conditioning, electric typewriters, and other background noises in an office can be stressful, especially for someone already overloaded by other demands or anxieties. Very modest noise pollution can also reduce sleep quality without the victims waking or knowing why they feel less rested.

Suspect that noise is contributing to your fatigue if you work in a noisy environment, if you feel better when noise levels are lower, or if you are easily startled or upset by noise.

You can reduce noise by using materials that absorb sound, including drapes, movable acoustical screens, acoustic tiles, carpets, and other sound-absorbing materials. In the office, noise can be reduced and personal privacy increased by rearranging traffic patterns. Computer-printer noises can be dampened by plastic covers. As a last resort wear earplugs or radio earphones.

Another approach is to mask noise with so-called white noise, a background hum containing all frequencies of sound. An air conditioner, fan, or certain forms of recorded sound can serve as white noise. Some experts advocate this approach. Others worry that white noise itself might contribute to stress. My personal choice is for classical music, which is soothing and a good noise-masker as well.

Climate and fatigue. Adverse weather conditions are an important, under-appreciated cause of chronic fatigue. As temperatures depart from the ideal range of sixty to seventy-five degrees, temperature stress increases. Health statistics reflect this in increasing death rates from heart disease and stroke.

Summer heat stress causes fatigue, particularly if stagnant wind, high humidity, or radiant heat sources such as the sun or an oven cause body heat to accumulate. Certain medicines reduce the ability to adapt to heat stress: major tranquilizers (such as Thorazine), tricyclic antidepressants, and certain antiulcer drugs.

Suspect excess warmth as the cause of fatigue if you often feel hot or if the temperature in your environment is above 80 degrees Fahrenheit. Air conditioning is the best preventive. A fan will work also, but only if the temperature remains below 90.

Cold stress can be difficult to recognize. As the air temperature falls below 60, body temperature also falls. One slows physically and mentally. This creates fatigue and vulnerability to accidents. Older people are especially susceptible. In England, where central heat is less common than in the U.S., cold stress is considered an important cause of hip fractures and other accidents among the elderly.

Drinking alcohol increases vulnerability to cold stress as does inadequate fluid intake (dehydration), malnutrition, hypoglycemia, hypothyroidism, and various medicines.

Suspect that cold stress is a problem if your room temperature is below 60 F. The best treatment is central heating. Next best is warm clothing or a portable heater. But beware of gas heaters or using an oven for heat. In addition to the risk of setting a fire, carbon monoxide poisoning is a real danger.

Sudden changes from warm to cold, as after a shower or going outdoors in winter, cause chilling, increase susceptibility to infections, and illness.

Humidity is a more important fatigue factor than many of us realize. Many of us lose energy and enthusiasm when humidity is high. Perspiration to cast off excess heat is less efficient. Mold counts, dust mite, some bacteria, and certain indoor air-pollutant levels increase (such as that of formaldehyde).

Low humidity also creates problems, among them itchy throat, dry cough, a chilly sensation, and increased vulnerability to infection. All can foster feelings of fatigue.

Individual comfort zones vary considerably, although most people are fine at relative humidities between 35 percent and 60 percent. You can purchase an inexpensive humidistat at most hardware stores. Use a humidifier to moisten the air or dehumidifiers, air conditioning, or forced air heating to dry it.

Air pressure (or barometric) changes also affect how we feel. Many persons with arthritis suffer during the period of low pressure that precedes a storm. Some feel sluggish when the barometer drops. We don't really understand why or what to do about it.

Outdoor air pollution, when severe, can cause fatigue and discomfort as well as more serious conditions such as pneumonia and heart attacks. Residents of Los Angeles who have suffered through heavy smog can testify to its debilitating effects. Less severe pollution can affect people with heart and lung disease. Healthy persons may also suffer some mild ill effects.

High altitude and fatigue. Many healthy persons visiting high altitude areas such as the Rocky Mountains, Alps, or Andes experience breathlessness and restlessness and feel tired and ill at ease during their first days of adjustment. Persons with heart or lung conditions or with severe anemia may never adjust well. University of Colorado researchers, noting a considerable exodus of older people from the high Rocky Mountain areas of Colorado, speculate that even the healthy elderly may feel suboptimal at high altitude. Such people should consider a vacation away from the mountains to see if they improve.

Electromagnetic radiation. Electrical and magnetic radiation is a controversial "pollutant." Several years ago, personnel at the U.S. embassy in Moscow reported unusual fatigue, headaches, and various illnesses. The cause suspected was the microwave electromagnetic radiation the Russians routinely beam into the embassy for the purpose of eavesdropping.

Many machines create moderately intense electromagnetic radiation, for example microwave ovens (especially if they leak), CB radios, walkie-talkies, electric blankets, color television sets, and video display terminals. Most American authorities do not believe that such exposures are a health problem. Exposure limits in the Soviet Union tend to be much stricter.

High energy fields such as those near high-voltage power lines, power generators, and television and radio transmitters might be a problem. At least five studies suggest that persons living close to such power sources have a higher-than-expected risk of cancer. Two studies found an increased rate of depression and suicide.

Air ion imbalance—the quantity of positive versus negative charges in the air—is another controversial possible cause of fatigue. There is a brisk business in ionizers for people who believe that negative ions can improve energy and mood. Some scientific evidence supports this viewpoint, but not enough to be convincing. I have not been impressed by the effect of negative ionizers on my patients who have tried them.

Hazards in the home. Your home is your castle but, in addition to the environmental problems already discussed, it may also play host to several other important causes of fatigue. If you feel worse at home than you do elsewhere (at work, outdoors, or on vacation), take a critical look at your home environment.

Allergies to dust, mold, and pet dander, which tend to be worse indoors, can result in fatigue along with typical allergy symptoms (itchy eyes, runny nose, respiratory difficulties). In contrast to the often dramatic onset of seasonal pollen allergy, year-round indoor allergens are often more subtle. Victims may not recognize the cause of their distress.

Suspect dust, mold, or pollen allergy if there are allergies in your family, if during the winter you are worse indoors, or if you have a frequent stuffed nose, post-nasal drip, or a perpetual cold. Allergy patients may feel worse after housecleaning, in moldy-damp basements, or after cuddling a pet. However, allergic reactions can be delayed for hours, so the relationship between an exposure and symptoms might not be obvious. Fortunately, skin allergy tests and blood tests for allergies (RAST tests) can usually identify your indoor allergies.

Indoor air pollution may be a problem if your breathing feels blocked and you feel tired or irritable in poorly ventilated areas, during air pollution alerts, or after exposure to tobacco smoke, detergents, perfume, pesticides, disinfectants, or air fresheners.

The most serious indoor air pollutant is carbon monoxide. This deadly poison forms from the incomplete burning of gas or oil from a furnace, cooking stove, or garaged automobile. Symptoms of carbon monoxide exposure include spaciness, headache, and fatigue. These should lessen rapidly after several hours away from the source. Your gas or oil company or the state environmental protection agency can measure the carbon monoxide level in your home.

Much more common as pollutants are other products of gas or oil burning such as nitrogen oxide. These irritating chemicals damage the nose, eyes, and lungs. General fatigue and irritability also occur. Any poorly vented gas- or oil-burning appliance can generate substantial indoor air pollution. Poorly vented fireplaces or wood-burning stoves produce different but equally harmful by-products. In Northern winters, if a house is closed tight, irritating petrochemical products are almost always higher indoors than outside.

Tobacco smoke is an even more serious hazard. If there is a smoker in the house and you have a post-nasal drip, runny nose, or itchy eyes, you should assume that tobacco irritation is part of your problem. If it is sufficiently severe, fatigue can be a by-product.

There has been much publicity about the potential harm of formaldehyde. Particle-board cabinets, urea-foam insulation, lower-grade plywood, new carpets, and foam-rubber carpet pads all leak formaldehyde to the indoor air. Some authorities believe this represents a significant source of air pollution in the home. However, most doubt that formaldehyde is often a problem except in special situations such as mobile homes, where very high levels can occur.

Suspect an indoor air pollution contribution to your symptoms if you feel better when you are outside for long periods or if you improve when the windows are open. One key to treatment and to prevention is good ventilation. In most areas outdoor air is cleaner than indoor air. Opening windows and venting appliances with exhaust fans can help. Unfortunately, good ventilation requires several turnovers of air every hour. This strains the heating budget in winter and the cooling budget in summer. Therefore, the other key treatment is to reduce your exposure to indoor air pollutants by curtailing its sources. Ban tobacco indoors or restrict it to one room that vents well to the outside. Check for leaking appliances; if the problem is severe you might even replace your gas kitchen appliances with electric ones. The best way to solve an indoor air pollution problem is by a combination of removing pollution sources and improving ventilation.

Hazards of the Office Environment

In addition to noise, lighting, and air quality, there are still other causes of fatigue in the modern office. After the home we spend more time at work than anywhere else. For many, the stress of work is their main source of fatigue. This includes not just the psychological stress of hostile supervisors, difficult work pace, or office politics, but the true physical stress of an unhealthful environment as well. The factory worker's exposure to toxic chemicals, dangerous machinery, or poor climate control is a recognized hazard that is now carefully regulated. However, we have only recently recognized the more subtle hazards of the office environment.

Personal computers and video display terminals may be the most fatigue-inducing work innovation since the assembly line. VDT workers have more fatigue, eyestrain, head/shoulder/neck aches, and general irritability than workers in similar jobs who did not use VDTs. One survey showed 74 percent of VDT workers complained of fatigue and 91 percent of eyestrain. At least ten million workers in the United States spend all or part of their day working at a display terminal.

And no wonder! Staring through glare at a flickering, slightly fuzzy image a foot and a half away is a sure prescription for tired eyes, aching muscles, and clouded mind. Many VDT users hunch forward or lean back, seeking to capture a view. Often chairs, handrests, and footrests are poorly fitted to worker comfort.

VDT workers are also subject to a form of psychological pressure reminiscent of early industrial assembly lines. Instead of monitoring productivity at the end of each day, supervisors can monitor keystrokes minute by minute. If the pace is forced for too long the worker will suffer fatigue and other signs of distress.

Computers and video screens emit several kinds of radiation, which has led to concern about inducing birth defects or premature birth in pregnant women. Reports of eye cataracts in VDT workers have also appeared. Research continues on these issues, but so far there is little firm evidence that VDT radiation actually causes these problems.

For many VDT workers a poorly designed work space and furniture is the main cause of fatigue. If you work on a VDT, check out your keyboard position, screen height, brightness and contrast, leg room, viewing distance, chair adjustment, and light levels to be sure they are comfortable. They should be adjustable too, since your needs may change frequently.

Recognize that VDT work is best done in relatively low light. A hood on the top of the VDT or a glare screen can help shield your eyes.

There should be a mandatory break away from the VDT for at least fifteen minutes every two hours if visual demands are moderate. There should be a ten-minute break every hour if visual demands are severe. This is the recommendation of the Federal National Institute of Occupational Safety and Health. Adequate break time is in the employer's interest as well as the employee's. Productivity suffers if the worker wears down. VDT workers should have a periodic test of eyes and vision.

Office workers are concerned about environmental quality. In a recent survey office workers identified their priorities as good lighting, a comfortable chair, good circulation of air, the right temperature and humidity, machines and reference materials within easy reach, the opportunity to stretch and move around, a place to work when you need to concentrate without distractions, not too much noise, a window, a place to go to relax. These can affect how you feel at work and at the end of the day.

How does your work environment rate in these categories?

PART 5

PHYSICAL DISORDERS THAT CAUSE FATIGUE

CHAPTER

14

PHYSICAL CAUSES OF FATIGUE

Physical Causes of Fatigue That Should be Apparent from a Standard Medical Examination

Can you be sure your doctor has done all the standard tests for the most common, detectable physical causes of fatigue? Remember, a typical visit to a family physician or internist lasts only ten to twenty minutes. If the complaint is "Doc, I feel tired all the time," most physicians take a brief history of the problem (when it started, when it occurs), perform a short physical examination, and order a standard set of laboratory tests.

These tests almost always include a complete blood count, and a blood-test battery called an SMA or SMAC (an abbreviation for the name of the machine that runs many tests on a single blood sample). Often, but not always, the physician also requests a thyroid blood test, blood sedimentation rate, analysis of urine, chest x-ray, electrocardiogram, and a breathing test to evaluate lung function.

The screening laboratory examination provides an extraordinary amount of information about most of the organs of the body. Physical causes of fatigue usually produce some abnormality on one or more of these tests. Therefore, as a patient, one of your most important tasks is to be sure your physician has obtained the pertinent screening tests and that he has adequately looked into any abnormality that appears.

Table 14.1 lists the specific screening tests of a typical evaluation for fatigue and the type of disease or condition they are designed to detect. Check these against the tests done on you. Your physician should welcome your interest and be pleased to explain which abnormalities are significant. (Certain small abnormalities may not be of practical importance.) The doctor might repeat certain tests to see if they change or to double-check the laboratory against error.

Unfortunately, some physical causes of fatigue are not discovered on these basic examinations. Even the diseases these tests usually detect

Table 14.1: STANDARD SCREENING TESTS AND CAUSES OF FATIGUE THEY ARE DESIGNED TO DETECT

Test	*Condition revealed*
Complete blood count (CBC):	
Hemoglobin/hematocrit	Anemia, polycythemia
White blood count	Infections, blood cancers, immune deficiency
SMA	
calcium	High or low calcium
phosphorous	Low phosphorous
BUN (blood urea nitrogen)	Abnormal kidney function, dehydration, internal bleeding, excessive tissue breakdown
Creatinine	Abnormal kidney function
SGOT, SGPT, GGTP, LDH	Liver disease (such as hepatitis)
Sugar (usually done fasting)	Diabetes mellitus, fasting hypoglycemia (different from the dietary hypoglycemia discussed in the nutrition section)
Albumin (a blood protein)	Malnutrition, liver disease, kidney disease
Globulin (a blood protein)	Certain immune system or blood disorders
Sodium (Na)	High or low blood sodium
Potassium (K)	High or low blood potassium
Carbon dioxide (CO_2)	Metabolic imbalance
Chloride (Cl)	Metabolic imbalance
Thyroid tests	
T3, T4, T7	Over- or underactive thyroid
TSH (thyroid stimulating hormone)	Early or mildly underactive thyroid
Sedimentation rate	A nonspecific indicator of various inflammatory processes including infections and immune disorders (Many older persons have relatively high sed rates without any illness.)
Urine analysis	Kidney disease, urine infections, diabetes (not as sensitive as the blood sugar test)
Electrocardiogram	Various forms of heart disease
Chest x-ray	Various lung or heart conditions
Lung function tests	Various lung or heart conditions

can be missed under certain circumstances. Therefore, do not absolutely conclude that there is nothing wrong physically if the tests all come up normal. For example, an overactive thyroid might not cause the usual elevations of the standard thyroid blood tests (called T3, T4, and T7). A special test known as a Free T3 may be needed. If you have the classical symptoms of hyperthyroidism (see Table 14.2) but are normal on

Table 14.2: COMMON SYMPTOMS OF HYPERTHYROIDISM (OVERACTIVE THYROID)

Nervousness/anxiety	Perspiration
Fatigue	Increased bowel movements
Emotional instability	Weight loss (often despite increased appetite)
Muscle weakness	Difficulty concentrating
Muscle tremors	Menstrual irregularity
Rapid or irregular heartbeat	Eye irritation or protruding eyes
Intolerance to heat	Thyroid swelling or tenderness in the lower neck

Table 14.3: COMMON SYMPTOMS OF HYPOTHYROIDISM (UNDERACTIVE THYROID)

Fatigue/lethargy	Husky voice
Weakness	Weight gain (often despite loss of appetite)
Dry or rough skin or hair	Joint aches, muscle cramps
Intolerance to cold	Shortness of breath
Depression	Slow heart rate
Difficulty concentrating	Constipation
Puffy hands or face	Mood or personality changes

standard thyroid blood tests, ask your doctor about a Free T3. Similarly, standard thyroid tests might not reveal an early low thyroid disorder. Instead a different blood test, TSH (thyroid stimulating hormone), may uncover the problem. If your symptoms suggest underactive thyroid (see Table 14.3), be sure your doctor also measures your TSH.

The most common physical causes of fatigue that are likely to be detected by a standard office examination and laboratory tests are anemia, infections, liver disease, kidney disease, thyroid disorders, diabetes, abnormalities of mineral and acid/base metabolism, certain cancers, and most heart and lung disorders.

Physical Conditions Which May Not Show on Standard Tests

Several diseases very easy to overlook unless your physician specifically thinks about them, questions you, or orders special laboratory tests include those that affect the body's endocrine regulatory glands.

Adrenal gland deficiency or Addison's disease is a rare but important cause of chronic fatigue. Many early cases of adrenal-gland failure are misdiagnosed as psychological. The key clue for suspecting adrenal-gland inadequacy is darkening of the skin, which occurs in about 90 percent of cases. President John F. Kennedy was probably the most famous victim of adrenal gland-failure. His "healthy" tan was probably the result of his disease.

Other typical symptoms include weakness, loss of appetite, nausea, stomach pain, salt craving, dizziness on standing up, low blood pressure, low blood sugar, low blood level of sodium, high blood level of potassium. However, early cases may have few symptoms other than chronic fatigue. Persons at high risk for adrenal failure include those who have taken a long course of adrenal steroid hormones (such as prednisone, decadron, medrol) and those with tuberculosis.

If one or more of the typical symptoms is present, your doctor should consider the possibility of adrenal-gland problems. You might be referred to an endocrinologist or your doctor might do an ACTH stimulation test, which detects whether your adrenals respond normally.

Addison's disease is fairly rare and should not be confused with the weak adrenal-gland syndrome that certain chiropractors diagnose with great frequency. Although I have tried to understand what these chiropractors mean by this diagnosis, I have been unable to. They certainly do not mean the same thing as physicians do when they describe an adrenal-gland disease.

Overactive adrenal glands can also cause fatigue. This leads to symptoms known as Cushing's syndrome: slowly developing muscle weakness, a moon-face facial puffiness, overweight (especially a "buffalo hump" on the back), increased facial hair, acne, stretch marks, easy bruising, mild high blood pressure, and a variety of mental and personality changes. If suggestive symptoms are present, a blood or urine measurement of adrenal hormone levels will lead to the diagnosis.

A different form of adrenal gland overactivity is called pheochromocytoma (or pheo, for short). Pheo causes an oversupply of another adrenal-gland hormone, adrenalin. This can trigger a full range of hyper symptoms that eventually lead to fatigue. The most dramatic symptoms are sudden attacks or paroxysms of headache, sweating, rapid or forceful heartbeat, palpitations, panic anxiety, fear of doom, nausea, abdominal or chest pain, vision disturbance, hot flashes, or a dramatic rise in blood pressure. Between attacks people with a pheo may feel well or may have chronic fatigue, sweating, weight loss, or high blood pressure. *If you have recurring attacks of hyper or anxiety symptoms, especially if your blood pressure rises, your doctor should make sure you do not have a pheochromocytoma.* Fortunately, a simple urine test will detect most cases and a blood test taken during an attack will find most of the rest.

Heart, Lung, and Circulatory Disorders

When we think of heart disease, we usually consider as typical symptoms chest pain, shortness of breath, fluid retention (edema), or palpitations (heartbeat irregularities). Actually, chronic fatigue can be one of heart disease's earliest warning signs, even before its more typical symptoms are prominent.

Most cases of heart, lung, or circulatory problems can be suspected from the standard history and physical examination, especially if it includes a chest x-ray, electrocardiogram, and lung-function tests. However, this is not always so. In such cases fatigue may be the critical clue that a serious problem is occurring. For example, angina pectoris (chest pain due to heart disease) or even the initial stages of a heart attack can be present with fatigue as the only obvious symptom. Irwin Cohen, a fifty-nine-year-old diabetic is a case in point.

Irwin keeps moderately fit slow-jogging two miles four times a week. For the last few months he has not felt like himself. He tires easily, especially after exercise. He has not had chest pain but has had a vague chest tightness that he assumes is from indigestion.

Irwin's physical examination, electrocardiogram, chest x-ray, and blood tests were normal, so he might easily be told there is nothing wrong or that he is just out of shape. But Irwin is of an age at which hardening of the heart arteries is fairly common. He also has one major risk factor for heart disease, diabetes. His fatigue therefore took on greater significance.

I asked Irwin to take a cardiac stress test, which is basically an electrocardiogram examination done while exercising. The result indicated that Irwin's heart muscle was straining.

A repeat stress test using a more sophisticated technique (a Thallium Stress Test) identified an area of poor heart muscle contraction. Cardiac catheterization showed a 90 percent block in the artery supplying that section of muscle. An operation bypassing the blocked artery restored normal blood flow. After a period of closely supervised exercise rehabilitation, Irwin fully recovered his stamina for exercise and his sense of well-being.

Irwin's serious heart condition could have led to a heart attack. I had ease, since Irwin exercised regularly without any chest pain. However, we now know that this type of "silent angina" is not at all rare. Fatigue, especially during or after exertion, can be an early warning sign.

Consider that your fatigue might relate to worsening heart disease if:

- Fatigue began recently (within weeks or months)
- You know you have heart disease
- You are fifty or older and have one or more major heart disease risk factors: pain or pressure in the chest, shoulder, neck, jaw, or arm that tends to occur with exercise or get better with rest; rapid, irregular, or unusually slow heartbeat; a family history of atherosclerosis, heart attack, or sudden death before age fifty-five; tobacco smoking; high blood pressure; high blood cholesterol; diabetes.

Abnormal heart valves. Another easily overlooked cause of tiredness is an abnormality of the heart's valves.

Melissa O'Brien is thirty-five. She has been feeling tired for about a year. Recently physical activity such as cleaning the house has left her weak and breathless.

She had a heart murmur as a child. However, when she first consulted her doctor about her fatigue a year ago, he could not hear a murmur. Now he hears a soft rumble, but only in an area the size of a quarter and only when she lies on her left side. Her chest x-ray had been read as normal last year. Now there is a subtle enlargement of one chamber of the heart. Mrs. O'Brien's electrocardiogram was also slightly abnormal, a change small enough to be easily missed. The doctor was not sure if there was a heart problem, so he ordered an echocardiogram, which creates a detailed image of the heart by measuring the echo of sound waves reflected from the inner structures of the heart.

Mrs. O'Brien's echocardiogram showed a narrowing or stenosis of the mitral valve, a tissue that separates the heart's small upper chamber from its muscular lower chamber. The narrow mitral valve partially blocked blood flow through the heart. This in turn reduced the volume of blood pumped to the body's tissues. With less oxygen and nutrients delivered to the tissues by the blood, Mrs. O'Brien's capacity for exertion decreased and the result was fatigue.

Although most forms of heart-valve disease are clearly signaled by the noise or murmur made by blood rushing over the deformed valve, certain heart-valve murmurs such as that of mitral stenosis can be extremely difficult to detect.

> Consider disease of the heart valves or other subtle heart conditions as a possible reason for your fatigue if:
>
> • You ever had a heart murmur, infection of the heart valve, rheumatic fever, or other heart disease
>
> • You suffer from shortness of breath, chest tightness or pain, chronic cough, coughing up blood, decreased ability to exercise, heart palpitations, lightheadedness, high or low blood pressure, or swollen ankles.

Blood clots. Blood clots in the heart-lung system can also present as unexplained fatigue.

Kathy Jordan, a cigarette smoker, is thirty-eight. She had become increasingly tired for several months. She felt breathless initially and more recently noted a decrease in her exercise capacity, occasional dizzy spells, lightheadedness, and anxiety.

Mrs. Jordan has taken birth control pills for twelve years. She did not stop despite an episode of blood clotting in the veins of one leg three years earlier.

At 3:00 A.M one Sunday, she woke in bed with excruciating chest pain, sweating, and shortness of breath. On the way to the hospital she began coughing blood.

In the emergency room an electrocardiogram showed no sign of a heart attack but indicated that her heart muscle was straining against an unusual load. Small patches appeared on Kathy Jordan's chest x-ray. An emergency scan of her lungs showed they had been damaged by blood clots.

Another procedure disclosed the source of the problem, a large blood clot in the vein of her upper leg. Pieces had broken off to lodge in her lung. Such clots are called pulmonary (lung) emboli. Probably smaller, painless clots had been bombarding her lung for several months, causing her fatigue, breathlessness, and lightheadedness. Unfortunately, the nervousness that accompanied her recent symptoms had led her doctor to focus on emotional rather than physical causes. Ironically, her nervousness was probably also the result of the physical impact of small pulmonary emboli.

In Mrs. Jordan's case the main villains were her birth control pills and cigarettes. Both increase the likelihood of blood clotting problems, especially among women past age thirty-five. Initially there was little to suggest pulmonary embolism as the cause of fatigue, although, in retrospect, the previous blood clot in her leg was a clue.

High blood pressure. High blood pressure can cause fatigue, headaches, and other symptoms. Therefore, your blood pressure should be checked as part of your general evaluation for fatigue. Nevertheless, it is also true that in most instances how you feel is not a reliable indicator of your blood pressure. You can feel well despite high blood pressure and feel miserable while your blood pressure is normal.

Congestive heart failure can result from untreated high blood pressure, viral infection of the heart muscle, or undetected valve disease. Fatigue is often prominent in congestive heart failure. However, shortness of breath or swelling of the feet usually provides the clue to look carefully at the heart.

Low blood pressure. A substantial minority of normal, healthy people have systolic blood pressures of 100, 90, or even less (the normal is 120). Usually, such low blood pressure is not a problem. Indeed, it might actually help to prevent a heart attack or stroke. However, in certain individuals low blood pressure reflects illness and can contribute to chronic fatigue.

Suspect that low blood pressure might be a problem if your current blood pressure is consistently below previous readings or if you become lightheaded when you first stand up, when you remain standing, or when you exercise. Medicines such as diuretics are the most common cause of symptomatic low blood pressure.

Your doctor can check for low blood pressure by measuring your blood pressure both lying down and standing up. A sharp drop on standing may indicate a problem. He might ask you to wear a portable blood pressure monitoring device, allowing an automatic check when your symptoms appear.

Some individuals have symptoms that mimic low blood pressure but with normal blood pressure readings. Recently, researchers at the Cleveland Clinic discovered that some of these individuals have an abnormally low volume of blood in their blood vessels. They believe this might be the reason for their fatigue, weakness, and dizziness. Were it not for this insight, no doubt, such patients' symptoms of fatigue and dizziness would probably have been dismissed as simply psychological.

Lung Diseases That Cause Fatigue

Fatigue or weakness can be a symptom of lung disease. Lung disease is more likely if there is also shortness of breath, chronic cough, wheezing, chest phlegm, blue pallor, ankle swelling, or huffing and puffing with mild exercise. Be extra-suspicious if you have been a cigarette smoker or have ever been told you have emphysema, recurring bronchitis, or bronchial asthma. Significant lung disease is probably not present if your symptoms do not worsen with exercise and you have none of the symptoms mentioned above.

The standard chest x-ray is abnormal in most but not all people with significant lung disease. Lung-function tests should also be done if lung disease is suspected. For these tests you blow hard into a bellows that measures the force and volume of your air flow. A simpler screen is for your physician to count the number of times you breathe each minute. However, if you are aware that breaths are being counted, self-consciousness alone can increase your respiratory rate.

WHAT DOES IT MEAN WHEN I CAN'T TAKE A FULL BREATH?

If your problem is mainly deep sighing or difficulty taking a full and satisfying deep breathe, lung disease such as asthma or emphysema can be the problem. However, often the problem is mainly a stress reaction. Stress can trigger incoordination of the diaphragm, the large muscle between the chest and the abdomen that acts like a bellows when we breath. If your lung functions test normal, consider this a clue that stress incoordination may be the problem. The treatment is learning to recognize signs of stress before breathing problems start, relaxation training, and breathing control.

The hyperventilation syndrome is another problem that can result from lung abnormalities or from stress. People who hyperventilate overbreathe to a degree that creates an imbalance of blood chemistry. This can cause a variety of symptoms—weird mental function, breathlessness, numbness and tingling of the hands, feet, or mouth, a cramping sensation in the hands, chest pains, heart palpitations, nervousness, lightheadedness, shakiness, and even fainting. If attacks are frequent fatigue almost always results.

Even small increases in the breathing rate, if prolonged, can trigger an attack. Hyperventilation may be common and so subtle that neither doctor nor patient notices the increased respiratory rate.

The best test for hyperventilation (measuring blood carbon dioxide levels during an attack) is usually not practical. An alternative is for your physician to lead you through three to four minutes of forced rapid breathing. A degree of lightheadedness is normal during this test. However, if you also become extremely spacey, tired, numb, or agitated or reproduce any other of your symptoms, hyperventilation is probably part of your problem.

If lung function is normal, stress is the most common reason for hyperventilation. However, many authorities believe (and I agree) that some people who hyperventilate probably have a metabolic or neurological abnormality that makes their breathing particularly vulnerable to hyperventilation.

Other conditions can mimic hyperventilation syndrome: an excess of acidity in the blood; pulmonary embolism, heart or lung disease, liver disease, low-blood-calcium or magnesium levels, head trauma, pain, panic disorder, and general anxiety.

Exercise and the Cardiovascular System

Both too much and too little exercise can cause fatigue.

Ginger Brown had been a high school athlete. Now at forty she was overweight and out of shape. Her husband Jack, a prominent chemist, faced his midlife crisis by becoming a marathon runner. He kept pushing Ginger to get in shape. She enrolled in an aerobics class, pushing hard for several months. To her surprise she felt worse after exercise instead of better. Fatigue, restlessness, and a vague ache in her muscles plagued her throughout the day.

I asked Ginger to measure her pulse during her aerobics workout. It was about 190, much higher than the target heart rate of 141 to 157 recommended for a forty-year-old's endurance training. After stopping exercise for one-minute her heart rate declined to 160, still higher than the one minute recovery target of 130 or less. Ginger was overexercising. When she slowed down her well-being improved.

Ginger's case shows that you can become overtired from exercising too much. Moderate exercise regularly is better than overdoing it. Table 14.4 provides typical recommendations for target heart rate for an exercise program.

> If you feel worse after you exercise, or if your exercise tolerance fails to improve after several months' training and a medical examination shows you are in good health, you may be overdoing your physical activity.

Some individuals feel profoundly lethargic if they do not obtain regular exercise. For many people, a steady exercise program can improve resistance to tiredness even when inactivity itself is not the main cause of fatigue. Part of exercise's benefit is from the strengthening and conditioning of the heart and skeletal muscles. Part is from exercise's calming and antidepressant effects. These calming effects may be as much biochemical as they are psychological.

> Unless fatigue is due to a severe physical illness, everyone who is tired should consider exercise training as a potential treatment. This is especially so if you have enjoyed exercise in the past.

The toughest part of an exercise program is getting started. A person who is out of shape may not notice improvement for several months. Therefore, consider a minimum treatment trial to be four forty-five-minute exercise sessions a week for at least six weeks.

Start with capable supervision. Programs at a Y are usually good. Commercial aerobic programs can be fine, too, but many go too fast for people who are older or out of shape.

Individual exercising can work well if you are medically healthy and know how to create a balanced program of warm-up, proper exertion, and warm-down. Don't push too hard and work out without fail. There are many excellent guidebooks. One favorite is Kenneth Cooper's *The New Aerobics* (New York: Bantam Books, 1970). It recognizes the special needs of persons who have not exercised recently.

For beginners, walking is best. Later, road bicycling, stationery bicycling, swimming, and jogging can be added. Exercise videotapes are useful, but choose one that builds slowly, like Debbie Reynolds' *Do It Debbie's Way,* Richard Simmons' *Silver Foxes,* Kathy Smith's *Body Basics* or *Women at Large* (especially designed for the overweight). Jane Fonda's *Prime Time* videotape is excellent. However, her other tapes that call for a more vigorous workout should not be attempted until you are in reasonable shape.

Unless you limit your exercise to walking, you should obtain a medical clearance. Many authorities recommend a stress electrocardiogram for anyone over forty who is starting to exercise. Others disagree, claiming a stress test is unnecessary if you have no history of heart trouble, no heart disease risk factors (high blood pressure, cigarette smoking, diabetes, high cholesterol, family history of early heart disease), no symptoms that are possibly heart-related (chest pain, dizzy spells, heart palpitations), and a normal medical exam.

I recommend a stress test to detect silent heart disease, and also because a stress test can measure your current exercise capacity. This shows how much exercise you can tolerate and begins a record of your progress.

Table 14.4: TARGET HEART RATE FOR EXERCISE TRAINING ACCORDING TO AGE

Age (years)	*Target Heart Rate Range** *(beats per minute)*
20-30	145-164
30-40	141-158
40-50	137-153
50-60	133-145
60-70	129-141

* The lower heart rate reflects the minimum intensity of exercise that will produce an increase in exercise endurance or training. The higher number is a limit on heart rate that is imposed for safety to prevent undue stress on the heart or muscles. A physician may choose to vary recommendations for specific individuals, depending on the results of their stress test, disease history, or medication.

Overweight: Being overweight predisposes to high blood pressure, diabetes, heart disease, and other conditions. Nevertheless stable, mild overweight does not cause fatigue. Gross overweight can make you tired, requiring more energy for ordinary movement, restricting breathing, and preventing restful sleep. Moderate overweight has an intermediate effect, which is worse if the weight gain is recent.

Table 14.5: 1983 METROPOLITIAN HEIGHT AND WEIGHT TABLES FOR MEN AND WOMEN ACCORDING TO FRAME, AGES 25-59

*Height (in shoes)***		Weight in Pounds (In indoor Clothing) *Small Frame*	*Medium Frame*	*Large Frame*
Feet	*Inches*		Men	
5	2	128-134	131-141	138-150
5	3	130-136	133-143	140-153
5	4	132-138	135-145	142-156
5	5	134-140	137-148	144-160
5	6	136-142	139-151	146-164
5	7	138-145	142-154	149-168
5	8	140-148	145-157	152-172
5	9	142-151	148-160	155-176
5	10	144-154	151-163	158-180
5	11	146-157	154-166	161-184
6	0	149-160	157-170	164-188
6	1	152-164	160-174	168-192
6	2	155-168	164-178	172-197
6	3	158-172	167-182	176-202
6	4	162-176	171-187	181-207
			Women	
4	10	102-111	109-121	118-131
4	11	103-113	111-123	120-134
5	0	104-115	113-126	122-137
5	1	106-118	115-129	125-140
5	2	108-121	118-132	128-143
5	3	111-124	121-135	131-147
5	4	114-127	124-138	134-151
5	5	117-130	127-141	137-155
5	6	120-133	130-144	140-159
5	7	123-136	133-147	143-163
5	8	126-139	136-150	146-167
5	9	129-142	139-153	149-170
5	10	132-145	142-156	152-173
5	11	135-148	145-159	155-176
6	0	138-151	148-162	158-179

* Indoor clothing weighing 5 pounds for men and 3 pounds for women.

** Shoes with 1-inch heels.

Source of basic data: *Build Study,* 1979, Society of Actuaries and Association of Life Insurance Medical Directors of America, 1980.

Metropolitan Life Insurance Company in 1979. It does not speak directly to the issue of fatigue but represents the weight classes that experienced the lowest death rates according to life insurance statistics. Consider this a rough and indirect guide to weights that are acceptable from a health viewpoint.

Weight gain is usually due to eating too much and exercising too little. Other causes include hypothyroidism, overactive adrenal glands (Cushing's syndrome), medication side effects, fluid retention due to heart, liver, or kidney disease, nicotine withdrawal (quitting smoking), anxiety, and depression.

If overweight is part of your problem, a sensible well-supervised diet to lose one to three pounds per week should improve your energy within a month or two.

Losing weight too rapidly can also be a cause of fatigue. Unbalanced or extremely low-calorie fad diets can make you tired and be dangerous to boot. Appetite-suppressant medicines can cause fatigue by overstimulation. These medicines may also cause a letdown when the medicine stops.

Loss of weight without deliberate dieting can be a clue to other diseases that can cause fatigue; they include diabetes, hyperthyroidism, depression, or drug abuse.

Hidden Infections

Fatigue can result from low-grade infection that is not recognized because there is no fever or only slight elevation at certain times of the day.

Hepatitis. Many individuals with a slow, smoldering liver inflammation (hepatitis) become profoundly tired but do not have fever or yellowing of skin (jaundice). Such liver disease can persist for months or even years although the standard laboratory examination should routinely detect it.

Infectious Mononucleosis. This infection causes tiredness, sore throat, and swollen lymph glands that can last for months. Once considered as a possibility, its presence can be confirmed by a simple blood test. Some experts believe that the Epstein-Barr virus, which is the cause of mono, can also cause a different and even more serious illness that can trigger fatigue lasting for years. This syndrome, the chronic Epstein-Barr virus syndrome, is discussed in Chapter 15.

AIDS (ACQUIRED IMMUNE DEFICIENCY SYNDROME)

AIDS, which may become the dominant medical fact of the twenty-first century, is not a cause of unrecognized chronic fatigue. Its victims have more spectacular symptoms, including fever, night sweats, weight loss, diarrhea, and infections. However, some who carry the AIDS virus without developing the deadly illness can suffer from fatigue and few other symptoms.

If you are in a group that is at high risk for AIDS—male homosexual, intravenous drug user, or the recipient of multiple blood transfusions between 1979 (when AIDS first appeared) and 1985 (when testing of blood donors became routine), consider a blood test for the HIV virus that is believed to cause AIDS. If, in addition, you have chronic fatigue and enlarged lymph glands in several parts of your body, a HIV blood test is especially important.

Hidden bacterial infections. Bacterial infections usually cause fever, chills, or pain in the area of infection. However, some bacterial infections have chronic low-grade symptoms that are easily ignored. Chronic fatigue can be the result.

The standard examination provides a clue if your white blood count or sedimentation rate is elevated. Check your temperature at night or any time you feel warm. Low-grade fever can be limited to the latter part of the day.

Table 14.6 lists the most common "hidden" infections, their symptoms, and the medical tests to detect them.

Allergies and Immune System Disorders

Anyone who has experienced the full bloom of spring or fall pollen allergy knows that its misery and fatigue can extend beyond itchy eyes and runny nose. Year-round allergy to dust, mold, or animal dander is more difficult to recognize, yet these allergens can be an important contributor to chronic fatigue.

A stuffed nose can make you tired, whether your congestion is due to

Table 14.6: NONVIRAL INFECTIONS THAT CAUSE FATIGUE AND ARE EASILY MISSED

Infection	*Typical Presentation**	*Subtle Presentation**	*Screening Diagnostic Tests*
Tuberculosis	Fever, night sweats, cough	Low-grade fever	Tuberculin skin test
Fungus	Fever, cough	Low-grade fever	Fungal skin test; chest x-ray
Nose/sinus	Green or yellow mucus, pain in the sinus area, fever, abnormal sinus x-ray	Chronic nasal stuffiness and post-nasal drip; sinus x-ray may be normal	Nasal smear, sinus x-ray, fiberoptic rhinoscopy, trial of antibiotics
Gum/teeth	Fever, painful gums	Mild ache in gums, sinus area or face	Dental exam
Heart valve	Hectic fever, chills, sweats, heart murmur	Low-grade or no fever, especially in elderly or if taking antibiotics; malaise; anemia	New or changed heart murmur; blood cultures
Prostate	Urinary frequency, urgency, burning, rectal pains	Same, only mild	Rectal examination; examination of prostate secretions
Urine	Urinary burning and frequency; sometimes low backache, fever	Mild urinary or pelvic-area discomfort	Urine analysis, urine culture
Female pelvis, uterus, or cervix	Fever, pelvic pain, vaginal discharge	Mild pelvic distress, vaginal discharge	Pelvic internal examination
Bone (osteomyelitis)	Fever, chills, local pain	Local soreness	X-ray, bone scan
Intestines	Diarrhea	Mimics irritable-bowel syndrome	Stool cultures for bacteria, stool examination for parasites

* Fatigue is often present with all these conditions and therefore is not listed individually for each infection.

allergy, infection, tobacco, air pollution, or a physical obstruction such as nasal polyps, enlarged adenoids, or a deviated septum. In one experiment researchers at the Mayo Clinic blocked the nostrils of healthy young men with Vaseline. Within a week all became tired or depressed. Nevertheless many people, including some physicians, fail to appreciate the important link between the nose and fatigue.

You can decide whether your congested nose is making you tired by treating it vigorously for a week, observing the effect on your fatigue. This means antibiotics if there is an infection, antihistamine/decongestant pills (ones that don't make you sleepy), decongestant nose drops, and perhaps a brief course of anti-inflammatory steroids. (Steroids are relatively safe when taken internally for *short* periods or by nasal spray for long periods. Decongestant nose drops or sprays are for short-term use only.)

Fatigue due to nasal congestion can be controlled by a combination of medicine, allergy treatments, and cleaning the environment. The state of the nose while sleeping is particularly important, since congestion at night can impair sleep quality.

How to identify your individual allergies is discussed in Chapter 13.

Immune system disorders: When the body becomes "allergic to itself." Most of us think of inflammatory diseases such as rheumatoid arthritis as confined to the joints. We assume that fatigue results from the wearying effect of pain, medicine side effects, or the disruption of sleep. That is part of the story. However, these so-called autoimmune (allergy-to-oneself) diseases affect the entire body. Fatigue is as much a part of the basic disease as the joint pain itself. Fortunately, medicines that control the joint inflammation also relieve the fatigue.

Classic rheumatoid arthritis is easy to recognize by the hot, painful, swollen joints. However, subtle autoimmune processes might have little joint swelling. Instead, tiredness, malaise, headaches, or muscle pain may be the most prominent symptoms.

Consider the possibility of an inflammatory autoimmune disorder if your fatigue is accompanied by joint pains or swelling, rashes, low-grade fever, or any combination of disturbing physical or mental symptoms for which no explanation has been found.

Usually (but not always) active autoimmune disease causes an abnormality of the sedimentation rate or related tests for inflammation such as the C Reactive Protein (CRP). This, together with suspicious symptoms, should cause your doctor to do additional evaluation, including a test for antinuclear antibody (ANA). Autoimmune disease that causes fatigue usually responds to anti-inflammatory medicines and a proper balance of exercise and rest.

Occult Cancer and Fatigue

People with cancer are often tired, no surprise to that. However, many cancer specialists believe that fatigue can be an early-warning signal of a hidden cancer. Fatigue may be especially predictive for cancer of such difficult-to-examine organs as the large bowel and pancreas.

A periodic cancer screening examination is in order even if you feel well. However, if you are forty-five or older and have been unusually fatigued for less than a year with no apparent cause, a thorough cancer detection examination should be considered—especially if you have a strong family history of cancer, recent changes in bowel habits, blood in stool, black or dark stool, weight loss, or loss of appetite.

A screening examination for bowel cancer should include a rectal examination, a chemical test of the stool for blood, and/or an examination of the large bowel with a flexible sigmoidoscope and/or barium enema X-ray. There is no simple screening test for early cancer of the pancreas. Diagnosis is difficult because early symptoms such as abdominal distress, gas, and bloating mimic other more common conditions such as irritable-bowel syndrome. At present, the best test for early detection is a computerized tomography (CT) scan of the abdomen.

Dizziness and Neurological Problems

Individuals who are chronically tired often have accompanying symptoms that raise suspicion of disease of the brain or nervous system—for example dizziness, difficulty concentrating, memory problems, numbness or tingling, coordination or balance problems, tremors or trembling, trouble remembering, blurry or double vision, muscle weakness, a new or worsening headache. In the back of the mind may be a special fear of early senility (Alzheimer's disease), multiple sclerosis, brain tumor, or stroke.

Among these only dizziness ranks as a common cause of fatigue. However, other neurological problems provoking fatigue do sometimes occur.

Dizziness. Feeling dizzy can be confused with feeling tired. Since dizziness has different meanings and can be difficult to describe, tiredness/dizziness problems are often misunderstood.

Feeling dizzy can mean (1) a sense of rotation or motion (vertigo), (2) a sensation of losing balance without spinning, (3) feeling about to faint or lose consciousness, (4) ill-defined lightheadedness or mental cloudiness.

True vertigo is the result of an abnormality in the balance centers of the inner ear or its nearby connections in the brain. There is a sensation that one's head or one's environment is moving. One may feel as if on a ship at sea. Nausea sometimes dominates to the point that the dizziness might be overlooked. If vertigo is chronic, usually an ear, nose, and throat specialist or a neurologist is the professional best qualified to evaluate and treat it. Feeling unbalanced but without true vertigo can result from neurological problems such as poor vision or damage to the nerves that transmit sensation to the brain from the legs. In this case a neurologist is the best person to see.

People who feel faint or lightheaded can have a neurological problem but usually do not. An extraordinary number of physical and psychological conditions can trigger these symptoms. The most common include hyperventilation syndrome; anxiety, depression, and stress-related problems; stroke and other neurological conditions; vision problems; endocrine problems; low blood pressure; heart-rhythm abnormalities and other forms of heart disease.

Resolving the dizziness usually also relieves the associated fatigue.

Headache. Frequent headaches leave people tired. On the other hand, often the same causes and conditions that trigger a headache are also reasons for recurring fatigue—among them poor posture (from hunching over at a video display terminal, perhaps), muscle tension, low-grade dental infections, nose or sinus infections, allergies, autoimmune disease, hypoglycemia, caffeine addiction, and depression. Similarly, frequent migraine causes fatigue, but migraine's key triggers—stress, alcohol, food intolerance, tobacco irritation, allergies—are reasons for fatigue in themselves.

If you have frequent headaches and tiredness, search for the causes of your headaches. They probably also cause your fatigue.

Muscle-Weakness Disorders. Most people who feel tired or weak have normal muscle strength and stamina. However, the possibility of nerve or muscle weakness should be considered if: your eyelids droop; you see double; you become tongue-tied after speaking a while; you have difficulty lifting objects that had previously been easy; your hands or arms tire after light exercise such as typing or washing dishes; you have to strain to hold your arms straight out for a full minute; you have difficulty rising from a chair without using your hands; you are unable to squat down and rise, even if someone helps you balance; you cannot rise on your heels or your toes; your muscles tire walking a slight hill or stairs before you become short of breath.

Inform your physician if you suspect muscle weakness. Among the nerve and muscle problems that might be considered are medicine side effects (as from cortisone), thyroid disease, diabetes, alcoholism, adrenal disease, vitamin deficiency, syphilis, autoimmune disease, among others. Myasthenia gravis is a rare but important neuromuscular disease that often presents itself as fatigue and weakness.

Abnormal sensation and coordination. Damage to the nerves of sensation does not by itself cause fatigue. However, many of the conditions that cause nerve damage are also fatigue triggers. Odd sensations in the hands and feet (paresthesia) are frequently from nonneurological causes such as hyperventilation or anxiety. You need a neurological exam by a doctor to be sure.

If you have trouble distinguishing a penny from a quarter, a sharp pin from a dull object, walking a straight line, keeping your balance when your eyes are closed (Don't try this by yourself!) or making rapid repetitive movements with your hands or feet, suspect possible damage to sensory nerves or to the centers of coordination. *Multiple sclerosis* can masquerade as almost any neurological disorder, causing temporary weakness, odd sensations, coordination difficulties, or mental abnormalities. Often fatigue is a prominent symptom. MS is a relatively uncommon disorder that was until recently difficult to exclude with certainty. Now special nerve conduction tests and an extremely sensitive imaging technique, nuclear magnetic resonance (NMR) can tell reliably whether multiple sclerosis is present.

Memory Problems. Early senility or Alzheimer's disease is probably the most feared diagnosis among older people who are tired and find their concentration failing. Although many Alzheimer's victims develop fatigue and/or depression, the vast majority of tired forgetful persons are not becoming senile. Most often their symptoms are results of distraction, worry or anxiety, or the side effects of a medicine or another physical illness. The physician can usually make a fair estimate of whether there is genuine memory failure. If he is not sure, he would request an evaluation by a neurologist.

CHAPTER

15

CONTROVERSIAL PHYSICAL CAUSES OF FATIGUE

This chapter discusses potentially important causes of fatigue that are not fully accepted by medical authorities. These may be important (I think most probably are) but for now they should be approached with appropriate caution.

Did your chronic fatigue first begin or become worse after a cold, an intestinal virus, or a bout with the flu? Do you feel as if you have a perpetual virus infection—stuffy nose, muscle aches, sore throat, swollen glands, low-grade fever, night sweats? If so, could you be hosting a deep-seated virus that is making you ill?

T.J. was a twenty-six-year-old physician just beginning his career when he contracted chicken pox. From then on he never felt well. He was always tired, especially after mild exercise or mental concentration. His symptoms were so draining he had to stop practicing medicine.

All in his head? One would hardly blame his doctors for thinking so, since a young physician's work can be stressful. Fortunately, they took T.J.'s story at face value and sought a link between his symptoms and his initial chicken-pox infection.

To test this theory, T.J.'s doctors used a nuclear magnetic resonance machine, a remarkable device that looks inside a living cell to read its biochemistry. They asked him to squeeze a rubber ball while holding his forearm in the field of the NMR. Exercise beyond a muscle's capacity increases the acid content within that muscle. Sure enough, acid within T.J's forearm muscle increased much more rapidly than it should in a healthy person.

T.J's muscle fatigue was not psychological. His muscle's chemistry was definitely abnormal, perhaps a persisting effect from the chicken-pox virus. We are not yet certain, but many researchers believe that a persisting virus infection might be an important reason for chronic fatigue.

The Epstein-Barr Virus Syndrome

The Epstein-Barr (E-B) virus causes infectious mononucleosis. A few mono victims never seem to recover or fall back periodically into fatigue, muscle aches, and other viruslike symptoms. As the science of immunology advanced into the 1980s, we learned that such individuals often had subtle abnormalities in their immune system's response to the Epstein-Barr virus; its pattern suggested a persisting infection with the virus.

There is legitimate skepticism about this interpretation. However, many scientists accept the view that chronic Epstein-Barr virus infection might be an important physical cause of chronic fatigue.

WHAT ARE THE SYMPTOMS OF CHRONIC E-B VIRUS SYNDROME?

Dr. Steven Straus of the National Institutes of Health identified twenty-two individuals whose immune-system profile suggested a chronic E-B virus problem. Essentially, all had continuous or intermittent fatigue. Most had mild low-grade fever, so mild it might easily be missed. Half reported frequent flulike symptoms (muscle aches, joint aches, sore throat, tender lymph glands, headaches).

Dr. James Jones at Denver's National Jewish Hospital described thirty-nine patients with a similar pattern. Jones also noted depression in 70 percent and mental cloudiness or difficulty concentrating in half. This suggests that chronic E-B virus infection might be a cause of depression and decreased mental function.

Many chronic E-B virus patients do not have a clear history of infectious mononucleosis. The standard blood laboratory test for mono is usually negative. Therefore, while chronic E-B virus illness is similar to mono in some ways, in other ways it is different.

Only a few years ago arguing that a hidden virus was an important cause of chronic fatigue was considered close to quackery. What now makes this plausible is our increasing ability to measure sophisticated abnormalities of the immune system. Sophisticated Epstein-Barr virus antibody tests are now available in some medical laboratories and should soon be accessible to all.

WHAT CAN BE DONE FOR E-B VIRUS VICTIMS?

There are no proved effective treatments for the Epstein-Barr virus syndrome, although several potential treatments are being tested. Antihistamines such as Seldane, antidepressant medicines such as doxepin

(Sinequan, Ativan) and anti-inflammatory agents such as Feldane may provide relief from symptoms. Many experts share the view that a positive attitude is good medicine. Stress management, adequate sleep, good diet, optimistic attitude, and spiritual faith may be of value.

Suspect chronic Epstein-Barr virus syndrome if you have continuing or relapsing unexplained episodes of fatigue, especially with low-grade temperature elevation, recurring sore throat, swollen glands, and/or flulike muscle aches. A blood examination for Epstein-Barr virus antibodies can confirm or refute this suspicion. However, antibody levels fluctuate and diagnostic standards are not yet firm. Therefore repeat examinations may be needed.

Immunology science is advancing rapidly. We should know before long whether chronic E-B and other hidden-virus syndromes are genuine diseases. Effective treatment should follow soon after.

"Hidden" Low Thyroid

Thyroid hormone therapy has long been espoused as a general treatment for those who suffer from chronic fatigue—much to the chagrin of most endocrinologists.

Dr. Broda Barnes states in his book *Hypothyroidism: The Unsuspected Problem* that low thyroid afflicts as much as 40 percent of the population. He views it as the number-one cause of chronic fatigue.

Barnes studied many patients with fatigue and noted that a large proportion of them had relatively low early-morning body temperatures, often below 97.8° F. As is well known, low temperature is common in hypothyroidism (and in several other conditions). Barnes wondered if thyroid supplements might help these patients even though most had normal results on standard thyroid hormone blood tests.

He treated them with thyroid and claimed dramatic improvement in most. Unfortunately, in his enthusiasm Barnes neglected to control for the placebo effect. Instead, he proclaimed his discovery as a new miracle cure. So far none of Barnes' followers has published proper scientific studies testing his claims.

Most thyroid specialists believe that Barnes' successes are entirely due to placebo effect. Nevertheless, evidence is accumulating that there may be a limited truth to Barnes' concept of hidden hypothyroidism. Many individuals with fatigue and depression do show abnormalities on new, sophisticated tests of thyroid function—despite normal results on the standard T3, T4, and T7 examinations. Whether thyroid supplements actually help such individuals is now under study.

If you and your doctor decide to try thyroid supplements, several cautions are in order:

Thyroid hormone is relatively safe if properly supervised. However, *persons with any heart abnormality can be harmed even at relatively low doses.* In anyone, too much thyroid can create the equivalent of an overactive thyroid state. Some of Broda Barnes' disciples risk dangerous hyperthyroidism by continuing to increase the dose of thyroid supplements beyond the usual treatment range until the morning body temperature finally reaches 97.8. This practice is a sure prescription for trouble.

Three Muscle Irritability Syndromes

IRRITABLE-BOWEL SYNDROME—MORE THAN JUST BOWEL?

One third of American adults suffer from an irritable bowel (or spastic colon: abdominal cramps, gas, bloating, diarrhea, or constipation. However, irritable-bowel syndrome may be part of a broader irritability problem, one that might be an important reason for chronic fatigue.

British researchers found that people with irritable-bowel syndrome compared to those with normal bowel function had a much higher rate of chronic tiredness, urinary-tract irritation, muscle pain, painful sexual intercourse (women only), headache, nausea, difficulty swallowing, bad taste in the mouth, poor sleeping, and several other symptoms. They suggest that irritable-bowel syndrome is part of a more general irritability affecting muscles throughout the body. Although many irritable-bowel victims are stressed or feel anxious, others seem normal emotionally but still suffer fatigue and diffuse irritability.

Having treated hundreds of tired irritable-bowel victims, I agree that irritable bowel is a systemic rather than simply a bowel problem. Fatigue is part of the syndrome. Although stress is important, this is not simply a psychological disease.

Many irritable-bowel patients improve with antimuscle spasm medicines or a change in diet. Some benefit from psychotherapy. In our experience with difficult cases, the most effective treatment is a nonpsychiatric program of relaxation and stress management using techniques such as muscle relaxation exercises and self-hypnosis. Often we find that when the bowel improves, energy also returns.

FIBROMYALGIA/FIBROSITIS

Many people who wake up with muscle aches and stiffness also complain of chronic fatigue, disturbed sleep, and tender points in the muscles of the neck, shoulder, and back. They have a syndrome called fibromyalgia (myalgia means "pain") or fibrositis (itis means "inflammation"). It may be relatively common. Certain arthritis specialists diagnose it in 5 to 10 percent of their patients.

Like irritable-bowel syndrome, fibromyalgia is often written off as simply psychosomatic—in other words, mental. Orthopedic surgeons are especially reluctant to accept this diagnosis. However, arthritis specialists, physical medicine physicians, and physical therapists do diagnose and treat it.

Factors that bring out fibromyalgia include stress, poor posture, overwork, sudden weather changes, and depression. It can also be produced by a disturbance of sleep. Disrupting a specific portion of the sleep cycle, even for a single night, can produce the syndrome, including muscle aches, tender points, and fatigue.

Suspect that fibromyalgia contributes to your fatigue if you also have muscle aches, morning stiffness, or unsatisfying sleep and you test negative for other forms of muscle and joint disease. To confirm the diagnosis your doctor should check for tenderness at specific points over the muscles of the neck, shoulder, and back. One way to treat fibromyalgia is with medicines that restore proper sleep cycle. Very low doses of tricyclic antidepressant agents have this effect. Muscle relaxants may help, as do other pain-control medicines. Physical therapy methods can be useful, including acupuncture, heat, ice, massage, improving posture, and anesthetizing sensitive trigger points. Stress management, physical exercise, and psychotherapy all have their advocates in this treatment.

TEMPOROMANDIBULAR JOINT (TMJ) DYSFUNCTION

I recently saw a thirty-five-year-old woman who had six weeks of constant pain on the side of her head. Not surprisingly, she was also quite tired. Her jaw wiggled and clicked when she opened it wide. When she closed her mouth her upper teeth pushed forward over her receding chin. Her regular dentist said he didn't believe in this "nonsense" about jaw misalignment causing head pain and fatigue. A second dentist disagreed. He injected a local anesthetic at the angle of the jaw, and within five minutes her headache had vanished.

Normal chewing or the habit of grinding teeth can inflame or misalign the temporomandibular joint at the angle of the jaw. This can cause tightness, tension or pain that can be experienced as headache, neckache, facial pain, or pain in the ear. Fatigue results from the chronic tension and pain.

Unfortunately, TMJ problems have been promoted as a catch-all for symptoms having nothing to do with the jaw. This has caused skepticism about its actual role. However, most dentists agree that the TMJ syndrome can be a real cause of facial tension and pain.

An intriguing aspect of the TMJ syndrome is that psychological stress can be both a cause and an effect. Psychological stress triggers jaw-muscle tensing and grinding of teeth. TMJ muscle tension and pain themselves cause psychological distress, potentially initiating a further cycle of jaw-muscle tension.

Hormonal Theories of Fatigue

PREMENSTRUAL SYNDROME (PMS)

If your fatigue and related symptoms occur almost entirely during the second half of your menstrual cycle and relent after the first few days of your period, premenstrual syndrome may be responsible. Until recently PMS was considered to be either imaginary or psychological. Now most physicians feel it is real and related to hormones, although firm proof for this viewpoint has been slow to appear.

Treating PMS remains controversial. Table 15.1 lists current treatments. The list is long because none of the treatments works for everyone. Indeed, even the most popular ones have not been proved to better the 40% rate of improvement often found with placebos.

The key issue is to be sure your symptoms really fit the PMS pattern. Being tired all month with worsening before your period is not PMS. To evaluate your pattern keep a diary of your symptoms. Take a long sheet of paper and turn it sideways. Along the bottom mark off the number of days in your usual menstrual cycle. Day one is the first day of your menstrual bleeding. Along the left-hand margin list your main symptoms. Each day write a symptom score beside each symptom—zero for no problem, ten for terrible ones. Do this for three months and you should be certain whether your pattern is that of PMS.

The symptom diary also allows you to notice other factors that may be triggering your distress. One woman wrote "I feel better when my husband is away." Leave a row to write in important life events. If your diary shows a persisting PMS pattern, ask your physician about a referral to a doctor or clinic that treats PMS.

MENOPAUSE

Did your fatigue begin at about the time you stopped having your periods? Did it follow a hysterectomy, removal of your ovaries, or another operation affecting your pelvic organs? At menopause women cease to release an egg each month, no longer have a monthly menstrual flow, and reduce the production of estrogen and progesterone from the ovary, while increasing certain hormones from the pituitary gland. While menopause provides relief for sufferers from PMS, some women date the onset of their fatigue to this time of their life.

Female sex hormones affect mood and metabolism. For some, hormonal shifts might be a physical basis for postmenopausal fatigue. These hormonal changes are often accompanied by symbolic or practical stresses such as entering "senior years," losing the mother role as children leave home, or having to pay for the kids at college. We can

Table 15.1: TREATMENTS FOR PREMENSTRUAL SYNDROME

- *Diet/Rest/Exercise:* Adequate rest; daily exercise; restriction of caffeine and alcohol; restriction of sugar; restriction of salt.
- *Nutritional Supplements:* Vitamin B_6 (beware of overdosing!);– vitamin E; magnesium; calcium; evening primrose oil (or black currant oil).
- *Stress Reduction:* Relaxation therapies such as yoga, meditation, muscle relaxation, visual imagery, self-hypnosis; biofeedback; support groups; individual or marital counseling; spiritual counseling.
- *Psychotherapy:* Individual or group.
- *Drug and Hormone Treatments:* Aspirin, candida yeast treatment; birth control pills; diuretics; antidepressant medicines; lithium; calcium channel blocking drugs; bromocriptine; synthetic progesterone; natural progesterone; danazol (antiestrogen hormone).

measure the hormonal changes of menopause but not whether they cause your fatigue. If your fatigue began or worsened with menopause and you have had a good medical/psychological evaluation, it is reasonable to consider a trial of estrogen/progesterone hormone treatment.

This assumes there are no medical reasons not to give hormones. Ironically, many experts recommend hormone supplements for most women—tired or not—hoping to reduce the risk of heart disease and osteoporosis (thinning of the bone). However, hormones might increase the risk of certain cancers. Therefore treatment must be followed closely by your physician.

Mitral Valve Prolapse

Earlier, I discussed narrowed mitral valve of the heart as an easily overlooked physical cause of chronic fatigue. Mitral valve prolapse is another type of mitral valve problem. Its role as a cause of fatigue is subject to dispute. Five to 10 percent of healthy adults have a peculiarity of the heart called mitral valve prolapse. The mitral valve is normal except for a looseness or floppiness where the valve attaches to the inner wall of the heart. This looseness causes an odd click that can usually be heard with a stethoscope and sometimes also a heart murmur. An echocardiogram shows the prolapsing mitral valve taking on a peculiar billowing motion, like that of the sail of a ship.

The vast majority of people who have mitral valve prolapse are perfectly healthy. However, a small proportion have symptoms such as fatigue, dizziness, odd chest pains, shortness of breath, abnormal heart rhythm, anxiety, and poor tolerance for exercise.

Many physicians believe mitral valve prolapse causes these problems. Others feel that the fatigue and other complaints are coincidental. Some experts believe that a subtle biochemical abnormality might bring out both prolapse and disturbing symptoms. In fact, some people with fatigue, chest pain, anxiety, and mitral valve prolapse are unusually sensitive to certain effects of the hormone adrenalin. Whether this is the reason for their symptoms is not yet clear.

Anyone who has mitral valve prolapse as well as fatigue, palpitations, shortness of breath, or chest pains should consider a trial of beta blocker treatment. These drugs block certain effects of adrenalin. Unfortunately, fatigue is also a side effect of this class of drugs.

PART 6

IDENTIFYING THE CAUSES OF YOUR FATIGUE

CHAPTER

16

THE *"WHY AM I TIRED?"* HEALTH HISTORY FORM

There are so many potential causes of fatigue that your doctor is not likely to have enough time to consider them all, not unless your history is well organized so that the prime suspects stand out. Often a medical history taken in discussions with a physician is so long, complicated, and filled with false leads as to be discouraging to even the most conscientious physician. Lacking clear leads, the physician may fall back on extensive (and expensive) laboratory testing. However, such testing is not usually productive unless it is guided by an accurate and well-understood history. Answering questions in advance can save hours of doctor time and highlight the most relevant facts. Organization is the way to approach your fatigue problem.

I developed the *"Why Am I Tired?"* Health History Form to help me quickly grasp the essentials of each new patient's problem. (I use a slightly different version in the office and find it invaluable.) It may take you an hour or even two hours to complete, but it will save you costly time with your physician—time the doctor might not have at any price. More important, it will help both of you analyze your problem systematically and to identify the most promising leads.

Make one photocopy of the *"Why Am I Tired?"* Health History Form. Fill it out completely, marking a check or "yes" next to each positive answer and a question mark if you are not sure. Put the form aside. After a day or two reread it quickly. The overall pattern of your responses should bring your attention and certainly your doctor's to the priority problems. Certain questions are repeated. That's because the same symptoms can occur in several diseases. It's much easier if the doctor doesn't have to piece together too many answers from different places. Many of the questions won't apply to you. We need to cast a wide net to be sure we capture your problem.

Next, make one copy of the form for your files and share the original with your doctor. You should schedule a long visit (thirty to sixty minutes) to review it.

"Why Am I Tired?" HEALTH HISTORY FORM

Name ______________________________ Age ______ Sex ______

1. State and describe your main symptoms in approximate order of their importance to you.

____

____

2. List any other important symptoms or problems.

____

____

3. List all hospitalizations and operations, their reason and year.

____

____

4. List all current medicines by name or purpose and any other treatments. Don't forget medicines such as aspirin, birth control pills, and vitamin supplements or treatments such as allergy shots and chiropractor treatments.

____

____

5. Indicate the severity/importance of your most important problem (#1) and your two next most important problems (#2 and #3) by rating them on a scale of 0 to 10. Zero means that the problem is minimal. Ten means the problem is very severe or distressing.

PROBLEM #	NATURE OF PROBLEM	SEVERITY/IMPORTANCE RATING (0-10)
#1	______________	______
#2	______________	______
#3	______________	______

6. About when did your problem first begin or seriously worsen? Describe. ____

____

7. Has your problem worsened much in recent weeks or months?

____

8. On the average how often are your symptoms present? (All the time, twice a week, etc.) ______________________________

9. List all medicines, diets, or other treatments for your fatigue or related problems, their approximate dates, degree of success, and the reason for stopping.

MEDICINE/TREATMENT	APPROX. DATES	SUCCESS/WHY STOPPED
______________	______________	______________
______________	______________	______________
______________	______________	______________

10. In addition to tiredness are you troubled by any of the following symptoms? (x-mild, xx-moderate, xxx-severe). Where several are listed together circle the one(s) that apply.

shortness of breath, breathless, rapid breathing, sighing, difficulty getting full breath	________
genuine weakness of muscles	________
overall feeling of weakness with muscle strength maintained	________
reduced exercise capacity	________
daytime sleepiness	________
too little, disturbed, or unsatisfying sleep	________
waking up tired	________
depression/sadness, loss of interest in life or activities	________
anxiety/nervousness/irritability/stress	________
weight loss or gain	________
recurrent fever or infections	________
frequent headaches/nasal congestion	________
irritable or upset stomach or bowels	________
muscle or joint aches	________

11. Do any other symptoms or problems improve or worsen as your fa-

tigue improves or worsens? (e.g., premenstrual symptoms, stress symptoms, digestive problems, nasal stuffiness)

____

____

12. What factors or situations tend to worsen symptoms (e.g., diet, stress, medicines, weather)?

____

____

13. What factors or situations improve your symptoms (e.g., medicines, more sleep, exercise, vacations, hobbies, diet)?

____

____

14. Is there a pattern to your symptoms? (time of day, day of the week, period of the month, season of the year, certain locations, indoors versus outdoors, weather changes, at home, at work, on vacation)

____

____

Specific Areas

15. Medicines and Drugs (see also question #9).

a. Have you and your physician specifically discussed whether your medicines might be contributing to fatigue? ______

b. Have you had any substantial period off each of your medicines since you developed fatigue? ______ If yes, did this "holiday" affect your symptoms? ______

c. Do you drink alcoholic beverages at least three times weekly? ______ If so, what do you usually drink and how much on an average day? _______________
Does drinking more or drinking less have any affect on your symptoms? Explain. _______________

____

Have you or anyone else ever been concerned that you might have a problem with alcohol? ______________________________

d. Do you take any medicine or drug at least once weekly to alter your mood or for recreation? For example: tranquilizers, sleeping pills, diet pills, marijuana, cocaine, heroin, glue sniffing?

____

e. Do you smoke tobacco regularly? ______________ How much? ______________ For how many years? ______________

16. Diet and Nutrition:

a. Do you feel that what you eat might influence your symptoms to a substantial degree? Explain ______________________________

____

b. Are you now or have you recently been on a special diet?

____

c. How many cups or glasses a day do you usually drink of coffee ________ decaffeinated coffee ________ tea ________ herbal tea ________ cola drinks ________ other soft drinks ________

d. Does drinking caffeine affect how you feel? Describe.

____

____

e. Does abstaining from caffeine or alcoholic beverages affect your symptoms in any way? ______________________________

____

f. During the last six months what is the maximum number of days in a row that you have taken no caffeine-containing products (e.g. coffee, tea, cola)? ______________________________

g. Does eating large quantities of high-sugar or high-carbohydrate foods or restricting these affect your symptoms?

____

h. Have you ever been told you have hypoglycemia, diabetes, or other sugar-related problem?

____

If you have had a glucose tolerance test, please obtain a copy of the result.

i. Are there other foods or diet patterns that affect how you feel?

____

HOW DO YOU FEEL WHEN:	BETTER	WORSE	SAME
skipping meals	______	______	______
extra large meals	______	______	______
high-fat foods	______	______	______
high-fiber or low-fiber foods	______	______	______
restaurant foods	______	______	______
chocolate	______	______	______
milk, dairy	______	______	______
food additives	______	______	______
fruit/vegetables	______	______	______
spices	______	______	______
other	______	______	______

Comments: ______________________________

j. Are there foods that make you feel good, or that you crave, or that you "couldn't live without"? ______________________________

____

k. If you currently or in the past took vitamins do you believe these influenced your symptoms? ______________________________

l. Which of the following foods do you eat?

	ALMOST DAILY, DAILY	2-3 TIMES A WEEK	LESS THAN WEEKLY
green vegetables	______	______	______
yellow vegetables	______	______	______
salad	______	______	______
margarine, vegetable oil, salad dressing	______	______	______

beef, lamb	______	______	______
chicken, turkey	______	______	______
fish	______	______	______
milk, butter, cheese	______	______	______
sugar, cookies, candy, ice cream, or other sweets	______	______	______
salt, salty foods	______	______	______
Others	______	______	______

m. Has it ever been suggested that you have a candida yeast problem? Describe? ____________________

Do you have:	YES	NO
frequent vaginal yeast infections?	____	____
frequent irritable-bowel or digestive disturbances?	____	____
a severe premenstrual syndrome?	____	____
improvement on a sugar/yeast restricted diet?	____	____
worsening with high-carbohydrate/high-yeast foods?	____	____
long exposure to antibiotics?	____	____
long exposure to steroid hormones (e.g. prednisone, medrol, cortisone)?	____	____
a history of taking birth control pills?	____	____

17. Physical Illness Overview:

a. Did you have a physical examination within six months or since you developed fatigue? (Note doctor's name/address/tel. #, and approximate date) ____________________

Did the doctor inform you of any problems or abnormalities?

____

b. Did the physical include:

	YES	NO	NOT SURE
blood pressure	______	______	______
heart/lung exam	______	______	______
abdominal exam	______	______	______
rectal/pelvic exam	______	______	______

c. Did laboratory tests include:

	NORMAL	ABNORMAL	NOT SURE	NOT DONE
Blood count (CBC-hemoglobin, hematocrit, white blood cell count)	______	______	______	______
SMA blood series	______	______	______	______
thyroid blood tests	______	______	______	______
sedimentation rate	______	______	______	______
urine analysis	______	______	______	______
chest x-ray	______	______	______	______
electrocardiogram (EKG)	______	______	______	______
lung function tests	______	______	______	______
Other tests (e.g., GI series, CT Scan, EEG)	______	______	______	______

18. Anemia (Check any signs that are present):

pale skin ______
pale under lower eyelid ______
heavy menstrual flow ______
poor diet ______
heavy alcohol intake ______
gastrointestinal diseases ______
malabsorption ______

19. Endocrine Problems (Check where the answer is Yes)

a. In your close family is there a history of:

thyroid problems ______
diabetes ______
other glandular disorders ______

b. Have you ever been told about any abnormality of your:

thyroid ______
adrenal glands ______
pancreas or sugar metabolism (e.g., diabetes) ______
pituitary ______
sex hormone or glands ______

c. Thyroid Symptoms:

feeling cold ________

feeling sluggish ________

frequent constipation ________

loss of eyebrow hair ________

feeling hyper ________

feeling warm ________

diarrhea ________

lump in lower neck or painful swelling ________

d. Adrenal:

darkening of skin ________

salt craving ________

dizzy when stand up ________

low blood sugar ________

round "moon face" ________

increased fat on chest or back ________

increased body hair ________

e. Unrecognized Diabetes:

frequent urination ________

increased thirst, or appetite ________

family history of diabetes ________

vaginal or skin yeast or fungus infections ________

foot infections ________

fluctuating or blurring vision ________

Have you had a recent blood sugar test? ________

Results: ____

f. Menstrual.

abnormal menstrual cycle or spotting ________

abnormal breast milk secretion ________

blurred or double vision ________

20. Heart, Lung, and Circulation (Check for Yes—circle appropriate answers):

a. Are you troubled by:

pain or pressure of your chest, arm, neck, or jaw, particularly with physical exertion ________

irregular, rapid, or unusually slow pulse or heartbeat ________

shortness of breath with minimal exertion: ________

climbing one flight of stairs ________

making bed ________

taking a shower ________

other ________

shortness of breath lying down ________

ankle swelling ________

b. Heart disease risk factors:

age 50+ ________

family history of early heart disease ________

high blood pressure ________

high cholesterol ________

diabetes ________

tobacco smoking ________

Type "A" personality ________

c. Have you ever had:

rheumatic fever ________

heart murmur or abnormal heart sound ________

mitral valve prolapse ________

abnormal stress test ________

abnormal chest x-ray ________

other abnormal heart test ________

d. Do you have:

chronic cough ________

rapid or difficult breathing ________

phlegm or mucous frequently, wheezing, asthma ________

wheezing, asthma ________

coughing up blood ________

pain in chest when you breathe ________

history of leg or pelvic vein inflammation (phlebitis) ________

blue lips or fingernails ________

work exposure to asbestos, heavy dust, irritants, or industrial chemicals ________

difficulty blowing out a candle or speaking for long periods ________

abnormal lung function tests ________

chronic bronchitis ________

emphysema ________

difficulty inhaling a full breath ________

hyperventilation syndrome: ________

- light-headed ________
- rapid breathing ________
- numbness or tingling of fingers or about mouth ________
- spasm or cramps of hands or forearms ________

e. Exercise:

Do you do vigorous exercise almost daily? ______ several times weekly? ______ Rarely? ______

Does exercise help ________ hurt ________ or not affect your symptoms? ______

f. Blood pressure:

Have you ever been told you had high blood pressure or taken a diuretic pill or other blood pressure medicine? ______

Do you often become lightheaded or dizzy when you stand up ______ or when you exercise? ______

g. Do you feel you are overweight ______ underweight ______ or about the right weight? ______

Have you gained ______ or lost ______ substantial weight recently or since you became fatigued? ______

Have you taken medicines to control your weight? ______ dieted strenuously? ______ induced vomiting or used laxatives to control your weight? ______

21. Hidden Infections (Check for Yes):

a. Do you often feel warm or have a low grade fever especially in the afternoon or evening? (If you haven't checked it, do so.) ________

b. Did your problems start or worsen at about the time you had a bad infection? ________

c. Do you feel as if you have a cold or the "flu" once a month or more? ________

d. Do you have symptoms or distress associated with:

nasal congestion or sinus infection ________

muscle or bone soreness or tenderness ________

urinary symptoms ________

a vaginal discharge ________

tooth or gum pain ________

frequent chills ________

abnormal sweating, especially at night ________

e. Have you ever had:

a heart murmur ________

hepatitis or exposure to hepatitis ________

possible exposure to AIDS ________

tuberculosis or an exposure to TB ________

f. Since you have been ill have you had:

a white blood cell count ________

a sedimentation rate or a C Reactive Protein (CRP test) ________

a urine analysis or culture for infection ________

a trial of treatment with antibiotics ________

a chest X-ray ________

sinus X-rays ________

a prostate examination ________

liver function tests ________

an internal (vaginal) examination ________

22. Gastrointestinal and Liver problems (Check for Yes.)

a. Have you ever been told you have:

irritable bowel or spastic colitis ________

gall bladder problems ________

ulcers ________

gastritis ________

esophageal inflammation (esophagitis) or reflux ________

liver disease or yellow jaundice ________

pancreas disease ________

ulcerative colitis or Crohn's disease ________

ameba or other parasites ________

b. Do you often have:

nausea ________

heartburn ________

belching, passing gas, abdominal bloating ________

stomach pain or abdominal cramps ________

diarrhea ________

constipation ________

blood in stool or black colored stool ________

recent weight loss ________

dark color urine ________

Have you recently had a change in bowel habits? ________

c. Have you had any stomach or bowel x-rays in recent years?

____

Results: ________________________________

(If abnormal, please obtain copy of report.)

23. Allergies and Nasal Congestion:

a. Have you had a frequent problem with:

allergies to pollen, dust, mold, or pets ________

nasal congestion, itching, runny nose, sneezing or post-nasal drip, snoring ________ itchy eyes, asthma, or eczema ________

seasonal variation in your symptoms ________

improvement or worsening when you are away from home for a week ________

unusual awareness of, or sensitivity to chemical smells such as: ________

tobacco ________

auto exhaust ________

fabric stores ________

gas range ________

soaps, perfume, air cleaner ________

newsprint ________

pesticides ________

b. Have you ever had allergy, skin, or blood tests? ________

Results: ________

24. Arthritis and Autoimmune Conditions:

joint pain or swelling ________

joint stiffness ________

unusual rashes or hives ________

fingers hurt or turn white in cold (Raynaud's phenomenon) ________

abnormal blood test for arthritis ________

abnormal x-ray for arthritis ________

25. Muscle or Blood Vessel Irritability Syndromes:

a. Irritable-Bowel Syndrome

abdominal gas or cramps, constipation or diarrhea with no other gastrointestinal disease being found ________

b. Fibromyalgia/Fibrositis:

muscle aches ________

muscle or joint stiffness (especially A.M.) ________

poor sleep ________

emotional distress ________

c. Migraine:

recurring severe headaches, especially if: ________

- on one side at a time ________
- preceded by warning symptoms or aura ________
- accompanied by nausea ________

d. Other Headaches Related To:

- stress ________
- posture/position ________
- nose/allergy ________
- medicines/caffeine/alcohol/foods ________
- waking you from sleep ________
- improvement with sleep ________
- worsening with sleep ________

e. Temporomandibular Joint Syndrome (TMJ):

- frequent pain in jaw, ear, neck, side of head, or behind eye ________
- abnormal jaw or tooth alignment ________
- worse with chewing, yawning ________
- jaw clicks when opens wide ________
- grinding teeth or tense jaw muscle ________
- pain radiates to ear, neck, side of head, or behind eye ________
- If you have frequent headache or pressure have you asked your dentist whether a tooth, gum, or jaw alignment problem might be relevant? ________

26. Hidden Cancer (especially of large bowel or pancreas):

- weight loss, appetite loss ________
- blood in stool, black stool ________
- stool abnormal on chemical testing for blood ________
- change in bowel habits ________
- anemia ________
- abdominal pain or distress ________
- family history of bowel cancer ________
- over age 40 ________

long-term alcohol use ________

long-term tobacco use ________

yellow eyes, skin, dark urine, jaundice ________

27. Diseases of the Muscles, Nerves, or Balance Centers:

a. Muscle weakness ________

difficulty lifting objects ________

difficulty rising from chair without using hands ________

leg weakness when climbing stairs ________

exercise tolerance reduced by weak muscle strength more than by shortness of breath ________

eyes tire if you blink rapidly ________

b. Coordination ________

feel unsteady ________

difficulty walking heel-toe on a straight line ________

tend to fall to one side ________

wide-based or unsteady walking gait ________

tend to drop objects ________

difficulty with rapid hand movement (e.g., typing) ________

tremor or trembling of fingers or hands ________

c. Abnormal sensation ________

numbness, tingling or pain in hands or feet ________

difficulty controlling urine/bladder function ________

difficulty controlling bowel movements ________

d. Mental status ________

worsening of concentration, mental judgment, memory, or reasoning ability ________

forget recent events while remembering distant ones ________

e. Dizziness/vertigo ________

sensation of motion/dizziness/vertigo ________

recurring nausea ________

loss of hearing ________

ringing in ears (tinnitus) ________

unsteady eye motion (nystagmus) ________

worse with sudden head movements ________

worse with car or other motion ________

tend to tilt or fall to one side ________

28. Stress/Anxiety

a. Do you feel nervous, jittery or anxious more often than you like?

____

b. Do you have some or all of the symptoms of anxiety described in Chapter 6? For example (circle those which apply):

Physical muscle tension or activity:
jumpiness, trembling, muscle tightness, heaviness or aching, fidgeting, restlessness, easy to startle

Symptoms of overactivation:
sweating, heart pounding, cold or clammy hands, dry mouth, lightheadedness, numbness, tingling, hot or cold spells, frequent urination, diarrhea, stomach discomfort, lump in throat, flushing, paleness, breathlessness

Fears:
worry, apprehension or fearful expectations about self or family, fear of losing control, fainting or having an accident, specific phobias or fears (e.g., of being alone, being in open spaces, closed in spaces, automobiles rides, bridges, heights, etc.)

Hyperalertness:
overawareness or scanning for threats or troubles in your environment or in your body, feeling on edge, irritable, impatient, difficulty sleeping

c. Has there been a recent increase in stress in your life? ________

home ________

work ________

finances ________

health ________

other ________

Comments: ________________________________

d. Might long-standing chronic stresses be wearing you down?

____

physical ________
emotional ________
at home ________
at work ________
financial ________
sexual ________
health ________
other? ________

Comments: ______________________________________

e. Do disturbing thoughts, dreams, images, impulses, or actions occur frequently? ______________________________

f. Has there been major physical or emotional trauma any time in your life? ______________________________
for example:

loss of a loved one ________
divorce ________
physical abuse/violence ________
sexual abuse (e.g., rape or incest) ________
war experience ________
survival from a serious accident, operation, or disease ________

Comments: ______________________________________

g. Have you had unusual difficulty adjusting to life's "normal" stresses, for example:

as a teenager growing up ________
separating from home ________
finding loving adult relationships ________
maintaining friends and social activities ________
fulfilling career ambitions ________
financial comfort ________
sexual and personal intimacy ________

adjust to aging parents ________
adjustment to raising children ________
adjustment to children growing up ________
physical or mental illness setbacks ________
loss of spouse or loved ones ________
loss of friends ________
adjustment to retirement ________
stresses of aging ________
finding spiritual peace ________
"meaning" in life ________

h. Do your symptoms
worsen with stress ________
improve when things are calm ________

i. Have you had a vacation in the last six months or year?

____

Do your symptoms improve when you are away for a week or two or more?

____

j. Does physical exercise help you
feel better? ________
feel worse? ________
no effect? ________

k. Do relaxation exercises (Yoga, biofeedback, meditation, muscle relaxation) help? ________________

l. Have you ever taken tranquilizers (Valium, Librium, Miltown, Phenobarbital, Fiorinal Donnatal, etc.)? ________________
What effect did they have?

____

m. Do you ever have panic attacks where you become unexplainably afraid, shaky, nervous or feel you are choking? ________________

n. Have you ever consulted a psychologist, psychiatrist or counselor or been in therapy? Describe. ________________

____

29. Depression:

feel depressed/sad or blue ______
loss of interest in your usual activities ______
loss of appetite ______
increased appetite ______
less sleep, early morning waking ______
sleeping longer ______
weight loss ______
weight gain ______
feeling unworthy, guilty, like a failure ______
thoughts about suicide ______
important reverses in your personal, family, financial, or work life ______
increased use of alcohol, medicine, drugs, or caffeine ______
a strong history of depression in your family ______
Have you ever taken medicines for depression? ______
Name ______
Have you ever been hospitalized for depression? ______
Is there a regular or periodic quality to your tiredness or depression? ______
Are there periods when you are super-productive, euphoric, or manic? ______

30. Sleep Problems (Check those that apply):

About how many hours do you actually sleep most nights? ______ Do you have difficulty falling asleep? staying asleep? ______ Do you wake early in the morning? ______ Do you snore? ______, toss and turn? ______ cease breathing, snort, or struggle to breathe? ______

Does pain, discomfort, noise, or other specific factors make good sleep difficult for you? ______ Is your nose congested when you sleep? ______ Do you get shortness of breath, chest tightness, chest pain, heart palpitations, or heartburn at night? ______ Are you more comfortable sleeping on several pillows than lying flat? ______ How many times do you usually wake to urinate? ______

Do you usually feel tired when you wake in the morning? ______ Do you feel achy when you wake? ______ Do you take sleeping pills more than once a week? ______ Do you fall asleep inappropriately at home, work, or while driving? ______ Do you often take a nap? ______

Are you now sleeping substantially less or more than you used to, for example, when you were last feeling well? ______
Comments: ______________________________

____

(If you sleep fitfully, ask someone to observe your breathing pattern and movement for an hour while you sleep.)

31. Pavlovian Conditioning/Anticipatory Anxiety/Vicious Cycle Anxiety:

a. Did your problems begin or increase markedly after a major illness, stress, or accident? ______________________________

b. Do direct or indirect reminders of a difficult or traumatic episode or period tend to trigger your symptoms? ______________________________

c. Once your symptoms begin does fright or panic tend to make it worse? ______________________________

d. Do you spend time or energy anticipating or worrying about your next episode of symptoms or illness? ______________________________

e. Do you have a powerful or vividly imaginative mind, or creativity in art, music, dance, or literature? ______________________________

f. Are you able to produce interesting, compelling, or detailed fantasies, daydreams, or changes in your mood with mental imagery or thoughts? ______________________________

32. Somatoform Disorders:

a. Has your fatigue been an almost life-long problem (at least since your early twenties)? ______________________________

Can you recall about when it began and what was then going on in your life? ______________________________

b. Have you for many years had many kinds of health problems or symptoms for which medical treatments have not been effective or for which no satisfying explanation has been found? ______

c. Do you, your doctors, or your friends view you as a hypochondriac?

______

d. Do you have an intense fear or concern that you have or will develop cancer, heart disease, AIDS, or other illness? ______

33. Environmental Sources of Fatigue:

a. Do you feel much worse when it is:

hot	______
cold	______
humid, muggy	______
dry	______
low barometric pressure	______
before or during storms	______
smoggy, polluted	______
other weather conditions	______

b. Are you subjected to unusual, distracting, or disturbing noises at home or at work? ______

c. Are you often disturbed by, exposed to, or unusually sensitive to environmental chemicals or odors at work, at home, or outdoors? ______

d. Can you tell a difference between regular food and foods without additives or between regular foods and organic foods?

______

e. Is there a seasonal pattern to your moods? ______

For example, do you feel worse in the winter or when you have little sunlight exposure?	______
Does exposure to outdoor light help you feel better?	______
Do you feel better or worse in the spring or fall?	______
Does being indoors or outdoors make a difference?	______

f. Are there environmental stresses in relation to your work?

difficult posture __________
repetitive tasks __________
heavy work __________
poor lighting or glare __________
uncomfortable temperature __________
uncomfortable humidity __________
crowding __________
noise __________
tobacco __________
indoor air pollution __________
productivity pressure __________
video display terminal use __________
poor air circulation __________
lack of privacy __________
no place to relax __________
uncomfortable chair/desk/machinery __________

Comments: ____

g. Do many people where you work complain of unusual fatigue, irritability, nasal congestion, itchy eyes, or other symptoms? __________

h. Is ventilation a problem at home or at work? __________ Are you exposed to tobacco smoke? __________ poorly ventilated or leaky gas or oil utilities? __________ poorly ventilated fireplace or wood stove? __________ poorly ventilated copy machines or other chemical processes?__________ excessive dust/mold/animal dander? __________

APPENDICES

Appendix 1

TWO ANTIHYPOGLYCEMIA DIETS

The Classic Antihypoglycemia Diet: Low Sugar, Low Carbohydrate, High Protein

Developed with my excellent dietitian, Lorri B. Katz, M.A., R.D., this diet is intended for a three-week trial to decide whether an antihypoglycemia-style diet can improve your energy.

General principles:

1. Eat three modest meals and several snacks. Do not skip meals.

2. Adjust the quantity of food to your weight goals. The example below serves 1300 calories a day. To maintain weight, an average sedentary woman should increase portions by about 25 percent. The average sedentary man should increase by about 50 percent. Although weight control can be a nice fringe benefit, this is not the diet's main purpose.

3. Acceptable foods:

Protein sources: Lean meat, fish, shellfish, poultry, eggs, cheese, farmer cheese, cottage cheese, pot cheese. Best choice is fish.

Vegetables: Any and all green or yellow vegetables or other nonstarchy vegetables, such as cauliflower, pepper, tomato, green beans—fresh or frozen. Avoid packages with sugar, cream, or added sauces.

Fruit: Intake should be moderate, up to two fruits a day. Whole fruit is preferable to fruit juices. You may have apples, berries, grapefruit, melon, oranges, peaches, pears, plums. Use fresh fruit or fruit-packed in water without sugar added. Read labels. Avoid dried fruit or candied fruit. They are high in sugar.

CLASSIC ANTIHYPOGLYCEMIA DIET: LOW SUGAR, LOW CARBOHYDRATE, HIGH PROTEIN (1300 Calories)

	Breakfast	*Lunch*	*Dinner*	*Snacks*
Day 1	1 orange ⅔ c. wheatena 1 boiled egg	green salad 2 tsp. oil/vinegar 7 oz. tuna in water 1 sm. pita bread ½ cup raw broccoli	4 oz. chicken w/o skin ½ c. spaghetti ½ c. string beans	1 oz. peanuts 1 oz. chicken + veggies 1 oz. cheese
Day 2	½ grapefruit ⅔ c. oatmeal 1 poached egg	cucumber tomato salad 4 oz. salmon salad ½ English muffin	green salad ½ tsp. oil/vinegar 4 oz. lean steak ½ c. barley, onions, mushrooms	2 tbsp. peanut butter on celery + veggies 1 oz. tofu 1 oz. almonds
Day 3	⅔ c. strawberries ½ c. cottage cheese	½ cup coleslaw 4 oz. turkey 1 slice bread	6 oz. broiled fish 2 tsp. margarine ½ baked yam ½ c. zucchini	1 boiled egg 1 oz. turkey + veggies 1 oz. soybeans
Day 4	½ banana ⅔ c. cream of rice 2 tbsp. peanut butter	4 oz. chicken salad 1 sm. pita bread raw vegetables	4 oz. lean roast beef ½ c. ziti with tomato sauce 1 c. spinach	1 oz. sunflower seeds 1 oz. tofu 2 tbsp. peanut butter on celery + veggies
Day 5	1 apple ⅔ c. oatmeal 1 scrambled egg 2 tsp. margarine	green salad 4 oz. cottage cheese with chives 1 pear 4 crackers	4 oz. chicken stir fry with 1 c. Chinese vegetables ½ c. rice	1 oz. soybeans 1 oz. chicken + veggies 1 oz. sunflower seeds
Day 6	½ grapefruit ⅔ c. wheatena 1 oz. cheese	½ c. coleslaw 4 oz. hamburger 1 sm. pita bread	6 oz. broiled fish 1 c. asparagus 2 tsp. margarine ½ c. spaghetti	1 oz. peanuts 1 oz. tofu + veggies 1 oz. cheese
Day 7	1 tangerine 2-egg omelette 1 oz. farmer cheese 2 tsp. margarine	green salad 4 oz. shrimp salad ½ bagel	1 c. chili (beef and beans) ½ c. refried beans 1 c. broccoli	1 oz. pumpkin seeds 1 oz. turkey + veggies 1 oz. walnuts

Nuts and Seeds: These are good sources of protein and vegetable oil but high in calories. Use moderately if weight is a problem. Prefer unsalted.

Dairy: Milk is a high-carbohydrate food, although it is also an excellent source of protein. Allow up to 8 ounces daily or substitute plain yogurt (without sweetener). Cheese is a high-fat, moderately high-protein with relatively fewer carbohydrates.

Beverages: Water, weak tea, decaffeinated coffee, herbal tea, club soda, and limited amounts of unsweetened fruit juice. Do not drink any alcoholic beverages, regular coffee, strong tea, chocolate, cocoa drinks, or soda. You may use limited artificial sweetener (in your decaffeinated coffee, but not in soda). The sweetness of the artificial sweetener stimulates craving for sweets.

Starchy foods: Simple sugars are strictly forbidden, including cane or beet sugars, corn starch or syrup, molasses, honey. Bread is limited to two slices a day, or substitute one serving of pasta. You may have one serving of potatoes (prefer boiled), beans or peas, or a whole grain (rice, barley, and so on).

Cooking oil and spreads: If there is a cholesterol problem, prefer pure vegetable oil and tub margarine to butter.

Use freely or in customary amounts: Spices, clear broth, herbs and spices, unsweetened whole gelatin. Moderate salt is okay unless you have high blood pressure, fluid retention, or another problem for which your doctor has advised restriction.

4. Eat all the alloted vegetables, fruits, and whole grains. These are your main carbohydrate sources. Eating too little carbohydrate provokes weakness and fatigue. It can be dangerous. The sample 1300-calorie low-carbohydrate, high-protein diet provides 70 to 80 grams of carbohydrates daily.

5. There are three meals and two or three snacks, midmorning, midafternoon, and evening. Substitutions are permitted.

6. Because individuals' nutritional and metabolic needs vary, obtain your physician's approval before starting this diet.

High-Complex Carbohydrate, High-Fiber, Low-Sugar Antihypoglycemia Diet

General guidelines are as for the traditional antihypoglycemia diet: frequent modest-size meals, no sugar, frequent snacks, no coffee, no alco-

HIGH-COMPLEX CARBOHYDRATE, HIGH-FIBER, LOW-SUGAR ANTIHYPOGLYCEMIA DIET (1300 Calories)

	Breakfast	*Lunch*	*Dinner*	*Snacks*
Day 1	⅔ c. stawberries 1 c. wheatena	lentil soup chef salad with chickpeas, kidney beans, roast beef, cheese, boiled egg, 2 tsp. oil	1 c. chili (lean beef, kidney beans) ½ c. refried beans 1. c cauliflower	1 c. blueberries 1 oz. soybeans + veggies 1 oz. walnuts
Day 2	1 orange 1 c. All-Bran 3 oz. milk	split pea soup 3 oz. chicken salad	6 oz. sole 1 c. broccoli 1 yam 1 tsp. margarine	1 oz. pumpkin seeds 1 fruit + veggies 2 tbsp. peanut butter on celery
Day 3	½ c. grapefrut 1 c. whole grain cereal or puffed wheat 3 oz. milk	3-bean salad (yellow string beans, green string beans, red kidney beans) 3 oz. tuna salad	4 oz. chicken 1 c. asparagus 1 c. kasha (buckwheat)	3 cups popcorn 1 baked apple + veggies ½ c. peas
Day 4	1 tangerine 1 c. Grape-Nuts cereal 3 oz. milk	black bean soup 3 oz. shrimp salad	4-bean salad (yellow string beans, green string beans, red kidney beans, chick peas) 4 oz. salmon ½ c. brown rice 1 c. string beans	1 oz. soybeans 1 oz. mixed nuts + veggies 1 fruit
Day 5	½ banana ½ c. oatmeal bran cereal 3 oz. milk	1 c. chili ½ c. refried beans	4 oz. chicken stir fry (pea pods, broccoli, zucchini, cauliflower)	2 tbsp. peanut butter on celery + veggies ⅔ c. strawberries or 3 c. popcorn 1 c. plain yogurt
Day 6	1 apple 1 c. wheatena	Pasta e fagiole (pasta and beans) green salad 2 tsp. oil	6 oz. fish ½ c. barley 1 c. zucchini	1 tangerine 1 oz. shredded wheat cereal + veggies 1 oz. mixed nuts
Day 7	mushroom omelette (2 eggs)	3-bean salad 3 oz. salmon ½ cup coleslaw	4-bean salad 4 oz. lean flank steak corn on the cob	1 oz. whole grain cereal 1 baked apple + veggies 3 popcorn

hol. High-fiber complex carbohydrates such as beans, brown rice, bran, and vegetables are actively encouraged. Protein is moderate. Adapt portion sizes to your weight goal. The sample meal plan of 1300 calories will cause most adults to lose weight. (Developed with the assistance of Lorri B. Katz, M.A., R.D.)

Recipes for Antihypoglycemia Diets

CHILI

(makes approximately 8 portions)

Appropriate for either classic or high-carbohydrate version of antihypoglycemia diet.

- 3 tablespoons oil
- 1 large onion, minced
- 2 cloves garlic, minced
- 1 lb. chopped beef
- 2 cups water
- 8 oz. tomato sauce
- 2 cups canned tomatoes
- 1 16-oz. can kidney beans
- 1 green pepper, diced
- ½ teaspoon celery seed
- ¼ teaspoon cayenne
- 1 small bay leaf
- 2 tablespoons chili powder
- ⅛ teaspoon basil
- ¼ teaspoon red pepper

1. Heat oil in skillet; add the onion and garlic and sauté until golden brown. Add the meat and brown. Drain the fat.

2. Transfer the meat mixture to a large saucepan and add the remaining ingredients. Bring to a boil, reduce the heat and simmer, uncovered, until the sauce is thick as desired, or about one hour.

The next three recipes are appropriate for the high-complex carbohydrate version of the antihypoglycemia diet only.

PASTA E FAGIOLI (PASTA AND BEANS)

(makes approximately 6-8 portions)

- 2 tablespoons oil
- 1 16-oz. can light red kidney beans
- 2 16-oz. cans white cannellini beans
- 2 16-oz. cans whole tomatoes (reserve juice)
- 4 cups water
- 2 large onions, chopped
- 2 cloves garlic, chopped

- ½ red pepper, diced
- ½ green pepper, diced
- 2 medium carrots, sliced
- 1 teaspoon basil
- 1 teaspoon oregano
- ¼ teaspoon black pepper
- 1 bay leaf
- 8 oz. macaroni

1. Heat the oil in a skillet; add the onions, garlic, and peppers. Sauté until golden brown.

2. Add remaining ingredients except macaroni. Simmer on low flame for 20 minutes.

3. Add the macaroni and simmer until macaroni is done, approximately 45 minutes.

BLACK BEAN SOUP

(serves 8)

- 1 lb. dried black beans, washed and cleaned, but not soaked
- 3 quarts cold water
- 2 tablespoons oil
- 2 medium yellow onions, minced
- 2 cloves garlic, crushed
- 2 medium tomatoes, chopped
- ¾ teaspoon oregano
- ½ teaspoon crushed dried hot red chili peppers
- ¼ teaspoon thyme
- ⅛ teaspoon black pepper

1. Place beans and water in large kettle. Cover and simmer 1¼ to 1½ hours until almost tender.

2. Saute onions and garlic in skillet until golden brown. Stir in tomatoes, herbs, and spices.

3. When beans are almost tender, stir skillet mixture into large pot containing beans and simmer 1½ to 2 hours longer, until beans are mushy.

4. If desired, purée mixture by pressing through a fine sieve.

SPLIT PEA SOUP

(serves 8)

- 1 lb. dried green split peas
- 4 tablespoons barley
- 2½ quarts cold water
- ½ cup chopped leeks
- ½ cup chopped celery
- ½ cup chopped onion
- ½ bay leaf
- chopped dill and parsley
- 3 medium carrots, sliced

1. Rinse the peas under cold water to remove all foreign particles. Let stand overnight.

2. Bring split peas and barley and water to a boil. Add the remaining ingredients. Reduce heat and simmer approximately 2½ hours—stirring frequently.

3. If desired, strain the soup, puree in an electric blender, and return to water.

Appendix 2

ROTARY DIVERSIFIED DIET FOR DETECTING FOOD ALLERGY

Choose foods that do not seem to give you a problem. Initially avoid the most common problem foods: milk, wheat, yeast, alcohol, coffee. (If you take much caffeine, consider withdrawal from caffeine before anything else.) Select a broad variety of foods from each of the following food groups: meat protein (includes poultry, fish, eggs), fruit, vegetable, nuts, spices. Repeat the same food only once in four days. After you have established improvement or a "safe" diet for three rotations, introduce one suspect food to your four-day rotation. If it is well-tolerated, incorporate it into your rotation. If you seem to react adversely, confirm the reaction by testing it again four days later.

The sample is of the most restrictive type of rotation diet, which provides only one food per meal. This should be taken in very large amounts so that you are not hungry. Rotation diets containing two, three, or four foods per meal are available.

Obviously, you should check with your doctor before embarking on major diet changes. Any diet intended for more than a few weeks should be reviewed by a registered dietitian.

SAMPLE DIET A

	Day 1	*Day 2*	*Day 3*	*Day 4*
Breakfast	apples	oranges	melon	berries
Lunch	lima beans	carrots	peas	squash
Dinner	lamb or goat	salmon, tuna, or trout	duck or goose	pork
Snacks	walnuts, yam	sunflower seeds, broccoli	almonds, grapes	coconut, buckwheat (kasha)

SAMPLE DIET B				
	Day 1	*Day 2*	*Day 3*	*Day 4*
Breakfast	beef	lobster	millet	tuna
Lunch	avocadoes	Jerusalem artichokes	mangoes	bananas
Dinner	salmon	turkey	sole	pheasant
Snacks	spinach	taro root (poi)	pumpkin	sesame seeds

A clear discussion of the rotation diet concept is found in Natalie Golos and Frances Golbitz, *Coping With Your Allergies* (Simon & Schuster, New York, 1979).

A more detailed and entertaining discussion is the subject of Natalie Golos's *If This Is Tuesday It Must Be Chicken!* This can be purchased through the Human Ecology Research Foundation of the Southwest, c/o Environmental Health Center of Dallas, 8345 Walnut Hill Lane, Dallas, Texas 75231.

Appendix 3

RECOMMENDED DIETARY ALLOWANCES OF VITAMINS & MINERALS

Nutrients	*Males**		*Females***	
	Age 23-50	*Age 51+*	*Age 23-50*	*Age 51+*
Vitamin A	1000	1000	800	800
Vitamin D	5	5	10	10
Vitamin E	10	10	8	8
Vitamin C	60	60	60	60
Thiamin (B_1)	1.6	1.4	1.0	1.0
Riboflavin (B_2)	1.6	1.4	1.2	1.2
Niacin (B_3)	18	16	13	13
Pyridoxine (B_6)	2.2	2.2	2.0	2.0
Folic Acid	400	400	400	400
Vitamin B_{12}	3.0	3.0	3.0	3.0
Calcium	800	800	800	800
Phosphorous	800	800	800	800
Magnesium	350	350	300	300
Iron†	10	10	18	10
Zinc	15	15	15	15
Iodine	150	150	150	150
Vitamin K††	70-140	70-140	70-140	70-140
Biotin††	100-200	100-200	100-200	100-200
Pantothenic Acid††	4-7	4-7	4-7	4-7
Copper††	2-3	2-3	2-3	2-3
Manganese††	2.5-5.0	2.5-5.0	2.5-5.0	2.5-5.0
Fluoride††	1.5-2.5	1.5-2.5	1.5-2.5	1.5-2.5
Chromium††	50-200	50-200	50-200	50-200
Selenium††	50-200	50-200	50-200	50-200
Molybdenum††	0.15-0.5	0.15-0.5	0.15-0.5	0.115-0.5

* Units are micrograms for Vitamin D, Folic acid, B_{12}, Iodine, Vitamin K, Biotin, Chromium, and Selenium. Vitamin A is in micrograms of retinol equivalents. Vitamin E is in milligrams of alpha tocopherol equivalents. Other nutrients are in milligrams.

** Not applicable if pregnant or lactating—conditions that increase nutritional requirements.

† The higher iron requirement for women assumes that menstruation occurs.

†† For these nutrients there is less information on which to base allowances, so no formal RDA has been adopted. Instead, there is a more tentative estimate of "safe and adequate" daily dietary intakes.

Adapted from Recommended Dietary Allowances, 9th rev. ed. (Washington, D.C.: National Academy of Sciences, Washington, D.C. 1980.)

Appendix 4

STRESS MANAGEMENT EXERCISES

Exercise 1: Deep Breathing

First, learn to breathe with your diaphragm and abdominal muscles, not just with your chest. Start by breathing slowly and easily through your nostrils. As you complete each breath, gently contract your stomach muscles. This pushes out the last of the air. Next, inhale deeply; exhale slowly with calm control. Continue to breathe freely and easily. As you do place your hands and fingers over your upper abdomen, your thumbs resting on your lowest ribs. Inhale slowly and deeply—feel the abdomen expand as you breathe in. This allows the powerful muscle of the diaphragm to drop down, expanding the lower lobes of the lungs to fill them completely with air. Exhale slowly and feel the abdomen contract. Imagine that with each deep breath you are inflating a balloon in your stomach. With each long, deep breath out you are releasing the air.

You may wish to count to yourself as you breathe in: "one-one thousand" or say "inhale." As you exhale slowly count: "two-one thousand" or say "exhale" or "relax." Many people prefer the time for breathing out to be twice as long as for breathing in. You may pause at the end of inhalation for two or three seconds before your slow breath out.

Slow, deep breathing is one of the quickest ways to relax. Any time you feel tense, take a slow, full deep breath in. Pause, then exhale slowly and deeply. Continue slow, deep, and comfortable breathing at four or five complete cycles per minute (a full cycle every ten to fifteen seconds). With each deep breath allow yourself to become more and more relaxed. After about two minutes you may resume your normal calm breathing pattern, feeling refreshed; or you may choose to continue deep breathing to achieve even deeper stages of relaxation.

*Exercise 2: Creating Your "Relaxation Response"**

1. Pick a brief phrase or word to focus your attention on. The word may reflect your belief system (Hail Mary, Peace) or be a simple syllable.

---

* Adapted with permission from Dr. Herbert Benson's *Beyond the Relaxation Response* (New York: Avon, 1976).

2. Choose a comfortable position—lying, sitting, or standing.

3. Close your eyes gently.

4. Relax your muscles. Starting at the bottom with your feet and progressing up to your calves, thighs, and abdomen, relax the various muscle groups in your body. Loosen up your neck and shoulders, gently rolling your head around and shrugging your shoulders slightly. Stretch and then relax your arms and hands, then let them drape naturally into your lap. Avoid grasping your knees or legs or holding your hands tightly together.

5. Become aware of your breathing and focus in on your chosen word. Breathe slowly and naturally, without forcing your rhythm. Repeat your word silently on each out breath. If you have chosen an entire phrase (The Lord is my shepherd, for instance), silently repeat the entire phrase as you exhale.

6. Maintain a passive frame of mind, as if basking in the sun. As you silently repeat your personal phrase or prayer thoughts will come to you. Respond to them in a casual, unconcerned way. Do not concentrate on them. Do not try to force them out of your mind. Simply adopt a passive attitude and continue to focus on the repetition of your focus words. Feel at liberty to scratch an itch or move to maintain your comfort. The relaxation response will continue so long as you remain in a comfortable and passive pose and focus on your key phrase.

7. Continue for a set period of time, usually ten to twenty minutes. Allow yourself to feel about when the correct amount of time has passed. Don't stare at a clock.

Once your session is over, sit quietly but keep your eyes closed for a full minute or two. Stop repeating your focus phrase. Allow regular thoughts to enter consciousness again. Finally open your eyes and sit quietly for another minute or two. If you experience mild dizziness from standing up too quickly, this is not dangerous. It can be avoided by the slow readjustment just described.

8. Practice the technique twice every day. It is best done before eating or several hours after a meal. Because this exercise is energizing, you may not wish to do it just before sleep.

Exercise 3: Progressive Muscle Relaxation

This type of exercise was popularized by Dr. Edmond Jacobson, a pioneer in the study of mind-body relationships. Allow for an uninterrupted practice session of about twenty minutes.

Lie comfortably on a bed or coach.

Relax your body. Let your weight sink heavily into the bed. There is no need for effort. Simply allow it to happen.

After a few pleasant minutes, slowly stiffen the muscles in both arms, but don't move your arms or clench your fists. Keep them gently stiff for about ten seconds, then tighten just a little more for another ten seconds.

Note how your arms feel. There may be a dull, taut sensation. Some describe a mild soreness or tenderness. Learn to recognize these signs of tightened muscles and nervous system activation.

Now allow your arms to relax gradually. As the sensation of stiffness subsides, note the feeling of easing tension. Rest in the relaxed state for one or two minutes.

Repeat the entire procedure. Contract and hold for about thirty seconds, then relax gradually.

Repeat a third time. This time, after you tighten, continue to let your arms relax past the point you ordinarily call relaxation.

As you continue to practice, you will learn to recognize the earliest signs of muscle tension. Similarly, you will recognize the feeling of relaxation more clearly and distinctly. You will be able to distinguish between completely relaxed states and those in which some tension remains. As you become better and better at this skill, simply tensing and "letting go" will create greater and greater degrees of relaxation.

Eventually, you can discontinue the period of muscle contraction since you are now acquainted with what tension feels like. With practice, you'll be able to relax every muscle group completely, without effort.

As you gain skill in progressive relaxation of the arms, continue to other parts of your body, particularly parts which are the location of some tension. For example:

Raise your eyebrows, wrinkling your forehead. Hold for a minute. Notice the feeling of tension in the forehead muscles. Gradually let the forehead relax.

Close your eyelids tightly. Hold for thirty seconds. Observe the tension. Allow the eyelid muscles to relax. Hold for a while. Repeat until you feel all the tension is gone.

As before, you can eventually eliminate the initial tensing period.

Remember, you don't have to exert effort to relax. Simply allow it to happen. If certain muscles remain tense, there may be deep-seated tension, which requires more time. However, attempting to force relaxation only adds to the tension, which opposes our goals for this technique.

Appendix 5

FINDING YOURSELF ON THE LIFE CYCLE SPECTRUM: ASSESSING YOUR PSYCHOLOGICAL VULNERABILITY

The time line below notes the ages of adult life, roughly divided. The age divisions are below the line. Identifying letters are above.

Each question focuses on feelings and attitudes that are critical during one or more of the predictable transition periods or "crises" of adult psychological development. Circle all identifying letters that correspond to the life cycle periods for which the stated feeling or attitude was relevant. This will provide an overview of the issues and outcomes of your life-stage transitions.

Questions relating to positive feelings and attitudes have been listed first (1-14). However, it is normal, even essential also to experience the negative feelings and attitudes in questions 15-28. Ordinarily, the negative attitudes and feelings should not be so powerful or of such long duration that they dominate your life. To the degree that you identify more with the negative than the positive feelings and attitudes, you will probably be more vulnerable to stress, depression and fatigue. Counseling directed at these issues is likely to result in feeling better and to greater resistance to the stresses of living.

A	B	C	D	E	F	G
age 16-22	22-28	28-32	32-38	38-45	45-65	65+

1. I felt I know who I am and what is important to me. A B C D E F G

2. I had a healthy balance of work obligations (job or family) with personal growth and caring relationships with friends and family. A B C D E F G

3. I felt secure enough to be myself and not overconcerned about satisfying the expectations of others.	A B C D E F G
4. I felt energetic and optimistic.	A B C D E F G
5. I felt comfortable making decisions without my parents' advice or worrying what they would think.	A B C D E F G
6. I had a healthy balance of giving and taking in those relationships that were most important to me.	A B C D E F G
7. I felt secure that if I were in trouble there were people I could turn to for emotional support.	A B C D E F G
8. I had a good balance of work and play.	A B C D E F G
9. I could experience a mature, stable love relationship.	A B C D E F G
10. I could experience sexual pleasure and closeness.	A B C D E F G
11. I found pleasure in helping others.	A B C D E F G
12. I had finally put "all the pieces together."	A B C D E F G
13. I felt truly competent.	A B C D E F G
14. I felt in touch with myself in a spiritual sense.	A B C D E F G
15. I felt I was always right and those who disagreed were wrong.	A B C D E F G
16. I felt confused about my sexual values or behavior.	A B C D E F G
17. I was dogmatic and opinionated.	A B C D E F G
18. I was too yielding or unassertive for my own good.	A B C D E F G
19. I was obsessed with "getting ahead."	A B C D E F G

20. I felt unproductive or stagnant in my work.	A B C D E F G
21. I felt unproductive or stagnant in my close personal relationships.	A B C D E F G
22. I felt isolated or lonely.	A B C D E F G
23. I felt pessimistic or cynical.	A B C D E F G
24. I felt angry or hostile.	A B C D E F G
25. I was often anxious or depressed.	A B C D E F G
26. I began to feel old.	A B C D E F G
27. I sensed time was running out.	A B C D E F G
28. I began to fear death.	A B C D E F G

Appendix 6

IDENTIFYING THE FATIGUE-INDUCING POTENTIAL OF YOUR MEDICINES

There are two tables here. The first lists the 150 most popular prescription medicines alphabetically according to the name under which the prescriptions are written (usually the manufacturer's trademark or "brand" names). However, drugs are also prescribed under common or "generic" names. This can be confusing, since a single drug can be known by one generic name and also one or more different brand names. The second table lists the most popular prescription drugs alphabetically according to their generic names and provides the translation into the pertinent brand names.

First, look for your medicines on Table 1. If it is not listed, look for it on Table 2. If you find your drug on Table 2, look up its brand name equivalents on Table 1. If your medicines are not on either table or if you wish more detailed information, consult the references noted in Chapter 12.

Table 1: FATIGUE POTENTIAL FOR THE MOST COMMONLY USED PRESCRIPTION DRUGS

Drug Name	*Generic Content*	*Type of Drug*	*Fatigue Potential 0 = little fatigue 3 = much fatigue*
Acetaminophen with codeine	Same	Pain	2
Adapin	Doxepin	Antidepressant	3
Aldactazide	Spironolactone plus hydrochlorthiazide	Diuretic	0*
Aldomet	Methyldopa	High blood pressure	3*
Aldoril	Methyldopa plus hydrochlorthiazide	High blood pressure plus diuretic	3*, **
Alupent	Metaproternol	Anti-asthma	0†
Amitryptyline	Same	Antidepressant	3
Anaprox	Naproxen	Pain/anti-inflammatory	2
Antivert	Meclizine	Antinausea/motion sickness	3
Apresoline	Hydralazine	High blood pressure	0*
Atarax	Hyroxyzine	Antihistamine	3
Ativan	Lorazepam	Tranquilizer	3
Benadryl	Diphenhydramine	Antihistamine	3
Bentyl	Dicylomine	Gastrointestinal	1
Brethine	Terbutaline	Anti-asthma	0†
Calan	Verapamil	Calcium channel blocker	1*
Capoten	Captopril	High blood pressure	0*
Cardizem	Diltiazem	Calcium channel blocker	1*
Catapres	Clonidine	High blood pressure	3*
Centrax	Prazepam	Tranquilizer	3
Clinoril	Sulindac	Pain/anti-inflammatory	2

Drug Name	*Generic Content*	*Type of Drug*	*Fatigue Potential 0 = little fatigue 3 = much fatigue*
Cogentin	Benztropine mesylate	Anti-Parkinson's disease or other movement problems	1
Compazine	Prochlorperazine	Antinausea; major tranquilizer	3
Corgard	Nadolol	Beta blocker	3
Coumadin	Warfarin	Anticoagulant	0††
Dalmane	Flurazepam	Sleeping pill	3
Darvon-N	Propoxyphene	Pain	2
Demulen	Ethynodiol diacetate + ethinyl estradiol	Birth control pill	1
Desyrel	Trazodone	Antidepressant	3
Diabinese	Chlorpropamide	Antidiabetes	0
Dilantin	Phenytoin	Antiseizure	3
Dimetapp	Brompheniramine + phenylephrine + phenylpropanolamine	Antihistamine + decongestant	2
Dipyridamole	Dipyridamole	Heart medicine; anticoagulant	0
Dolobid	Diflunisal	Pain/anti-inflammatory	2
Donnatal	Phenobarbital + hyoscyamine + atropine + scopolamine	Gastrointestinal relaxation	2
Dyazide	Dyrenium + hydrochlorthiazide	High blood pressure	0*
Elavil	Amitryptyline	Antidepressant	3
Empirin with codeine	Aspirin + codeine	Pain + anti-inflammatory	2
Entex LA	Phenylpropanolamine + guaifenesin	Decongestant + expectorant	0†
Feldene	Piroxicam	Anti-inflammatory/pain	2
Fiorinal	Butalbital + aspirin + caffeine	Headache/tension/pain	3
Flexeril	Cyclobenzaprine	Muscle relaxant	3
Furosemide	Same	Diuretic	0*, **

Table 1: FATIGUE POTENTIAL FOR THE MOST COMMONLY USED PRESCRIPTION DRUGS (cont.)

Drug Name	*Generic Content*	*Type of Drug*	*Fatigue Potential 0 = little fatigue 3 = much fatigue*
Halcion	Triazolam	Sleeping pill	3
Haldol	Haloperidol	Major tranquilizer	3
Hydrochlorthiazide	Same	Diuretic	0*, **
Hydrodiuril	Same	Diuretic	0*, **
Hygroton	Chlorthalidone	Diuretic	0*, **
Imodium	Loperamide	Antidiarrhea	1
Inderal	Propranalol	Beta blocker	3
Inderide	Propranalol + hydrochlorthiazide	Beta blocker + diuretic	3
Indocin	Indomethacin	Anti-inflammatory/pain	2
Isoptin	Verapamil	Calcium channel blocker	1*
Isordil	Isorbide dinitrate	Anti-angina pectoris	0*
Klotrix	Potassium chloride	Potassium supplement	0
K-Lyte	Potassium bicarbonate + potassium citrate	Potassium supplement	0
K-Tab	Potassium chloride	Potassium supplement	0
Lanoxin	Digoxin	Heart medicine	1‡
Lasix	Furosemide	Diuretic	0*, **
Librax	Chlordiazepoxide + clidinium bromide	Tranquilizer + antispasmodic	3
Librium	Chlordiazepoxide	Tranquilizer	3
Loestrin FE	Norethindrone acetate + ethinyl estradiol	Birth control pill	1
Lomotil	Diphenoxylate + atropine	Antidiarrhea	2

Drug Name	*Generic Content*	*Type of Drug*	*Fatigue Potential 0 = little fatigue 3 = much fatigue*
Lo/ovral	Norgestral + ethinyl estradiol	Birth control pill	1
Lopurin	Allopurinol	Antigout; reduces blood uric acid	0
Maxzide	Triampterene + hydroclorthiazide	Diuretic	0*
Meclomen	Meclofenamate	Anti-inflammatory/pain	2
Medrol	Methyl prednisolone	Adrenal steriod hormone	1
Mellaril	Thioridazine	Major tranquilizer	3
Micro-K	Potassium chloride	Potassium supplement	0
Micronase	Glipizide	Antidiabetes	0
Ortho-Novum	Norethindrone + ethinyl estradiol	Birth control pill	1
Ovral	Norgestrel + ethinyl estradiol	Birth control pill	1
Parafon forte	Chlorzoxazone + acetaminophen	Pain/muscle relaxer	1
Percodan	Oxycodone + aspirin	Pain/narcotic	3
Percoset	Oxycodone + acetaminophen	Pain/narcotic	3
Phenergan	Promethazine	Antinausea/antihistamine	3
Phernagan with codeine	Promethazine + codeine	Antihistamine/cough	2
Phenobarbital	Same	Tranquilizer/sleeping pill	3
Prednisone	Same	Adrenal steriod hormone	1
Premarin	Conjugated estrogen	Estrogen hormone	1
Procan	Procainamide hydrochloride	Heart medicine	1
Procardia	Nifedipine	Calcium channel blocker	2*
Propine	Dipevefrin	Glaucoma medicine	0
Proventil	Albuterol	Anti-asthma	1†
Provera	Medroxyprogesterone	Progesterone hormone	1
Pyridium	Phenazopyridine	Urinary tract analgesic	0
Quinaglute	Quinidine gluconate	Heart	1

Table 1: FATIGUE POTENTIAL FOR THE MOST COMMONLY USED PRESCRIPTION DRUGS (cont.)

Drug Name	*Generic Content*	*Type of Drug*	*Fatigue Potential 0 = little fatigue 3 = much fatigue*
Reglan	Metoclorpropamide	Gastro-intestinal	2
Restoril	Temazepam	Sleeping pill	3
Ritalin	Methylphenidate	Central nervous system stimulant	2†
Rondec-DM	Carboxinamine maleate + pseudoephedrine + dextromethorphan	Antihistamine, decongestant, anti-cough	1
Rufen	Ibuprofen	Anti-inflammatory/pain	2
Seldane	Terfenadine	Antihistamine	0
Serax	Oxazepam	Tranquilizer	3
Sinequan	Doxepin	Antidepressant	3
Sinemet	Carbidopa-levodopa	Anti-Parkinson's Disease	1
Slow-K	Potassium chloride	Potassium supplement	0
Slo-Phyllin	theophylline	Anti-asthma	1†
Synalgos-DC	Dihydrocodeine bitartrate + aspirin + caffeine	Pain	2
Synthroid	Levothyroxine	Thyroid hormone	0†
Tagamet	Cimetidine	Reduce stomach acid	1
Talwin Nx	Pentazocine + naloxone	Pain	3
Tavist-D	Clemastine fumarate + phenylpropanolamine	Antihistamine + decongestant	1
Tegretol	Carbamazepine	Anti-epilepsy	2
Tenormin	Atenolol	Beta blocker	2
Theo-Dur	Theophylline	Anti-asthma	1†
Thyroid	Same	Thyroid hormone	0

Drug Name	*Generic Content*	*Type of Drug*	*Fatigue Potential 0 = little fatigue 3 = much fatigue*
Tolectin	Tolmetin	Anti-inflammatory/pain	2
Tolinase	Tolazamide	Diabetic	0
Transderm-Nitro	Nitroglycerin	Anti-angina	0*
Tranxene	Clorazepate	Tranquilizer	3
Trental	Pentoxifylline	Improves blood flow	0
Triavil	Perphenazine + amitryptiline	Tranquilizer + anti-depressant	3
Trinalin	Azatadine + pseudoephedrine	Antihistamine + decongestant	2
Triphasil	Levonorgestrel + ethinyl estradiol	Birth control pill	1
Tussi-Organidin	Iodinated glycerol + codeine	Expectorant + anticough	1
Tylenol with codeine	Acetaminophen + codeine	Pain	2
Valium	Diazepam	Tranquilizer	3
Vasotec	Enalapril	High blood pressure	0*
Ventolin	Albuterol	Anti-asthma	1†
Vicoden	Hydrocodone bitartrate + acetaminophen	Pain + cough suppressant	2
Xanax	Alprazalom	Antidepressant + tranquilizer	3
Zantac	Ranitidine	Inhibits stomach acid	1
Zyloprim	Allopurinol	Lowers blood uric acid level	0

* Can cause low blood pressure, which in turn promotes fatigue.

** Can cause low potassium, which causes fatigue.

† Causes overstimulation, which can lead to fatigue.

†† Can cause internal bleeding, which can result in fatigue.

‡ Overdose can cause fatigue, depression.

Table 2: GENERIC NAMES OF PRESCRIPTION DRUGS AND THEIR COMMONLY USED BRAND-NAME EQUIVALENTS*

Generic Name	*Brand Name*
albuterol	Proventil, Ventolin
allopurinol	Lopurin, Zyloprim
alprazalom	Xanax
amitryptyline	Elavil (Endep, Limbitrol, Triavil)
atenolol	Tenormin
benztropine	Cogentin
captopril	Capoten
carbamazepine	Tegretol
chlorazepate	Tranxene
chlordiazepoxide	Librium
chlorpropamide	Diabinese
cimetidine	Tagamet
clonidine	Catapres
cyclobenzaprine	Flexeril
diazepam	Valium
dicyclomine	Bentyl
digoxin	Lanoxin
diltiazem	Cardiozem
diphenhydramine	Benadryl
dipivefrin	Propine
doxepin	Adapin, Sinequan
flurazepam	Dalmane
glyburide	Micronase,(Diabeta)
haloperidol	Haldol
hydralazine	Apresoline
hydroxyzine	Atarax (Vistaril)
ibuprofen	Motrin, Rufen (Advil)
indomethacin	Indocin
isorbide trinitrate	Isordil (Iso Bid, Sorate, Sorbitrate)
levothyroxine	Synthroid
lorazepam	Ativan
loperamide	Imodium
meclizine	Antivert (Bonine)
medroxyprogesterone	Provera
metaproternol	Alupent
methyldopa	Aldomet
methylphenidate	Ritalin
methylprednisolone	Medrol

Table 2: GENERIC NAMES OF PRESCRIPTION DRUGS AND THEIR COMMONLY USED BRAND-NAME EQUIVALENTS* (cont.)

Generic Name	*Brand Name*
metochlorpropamide	Reglan
metoprolol	Lopressor
nadolol	Corgard
naproxen	Anaprox,Naprosyn
nicotine	Nicorette
nifedipine	Procardia
oxazepam	Serax
pentoxifylline	Trental
potassium chloride	Klotrix, K-tab, Micro-K, Slow-K
prazepam	Centrax
prazocin	Minipress
prochlorperazine	Compazine
promethazine	Phenergan (Remsed)
propoxyphene	Darvon
propranalol	Inderal
quinidine gluconate	Quiniglute
ranitidine	Zantac
sulindac	Clinoril
temazepam	Restoril
terbutaline	Brethine (Bricanyl)
terfenadine	Seldane
thioridazine	Mellaril
tolazamide	Tolinase
tolmetin	Tolectin
triazolam	Dalmane
verapamil	Calan, Isoptin
warfarin	Coumadin

* Brand names in parentheses are less commonly prescribed and therefore are not listed in Table 1.

Appendix 7

CENTERS FOR THE EVALUATION OF SLEEP DISORDERS

Although individual physicians throughout the country are knowledgeable in sleep problems, particularly insomnia, difficult sleep-related problems are best evaluated in a formally organized center. The best centers are usually those affiliated with the Association of Sleep Disorders Centers (604 Second St. SW, Rochester, Minn. 55902). The following centers were accredited by the Association of Sleep Disorder Centers as of January 1, 1987. Sleep studies is a rapidly growing field, so there should be additional centers by the time you read this. If there is no listing near you, you or your doctor should contact the association directly. Centers whose names are followed by a (P) were provisional members in 1987.

ALABAMA

Sleep Disorders Center of Alabama
affiliated with Baptist Medical Center
800 Montclair Rd.
Birmingham 35213
205-592-5650

Sleep/Wake Disorders Center
University of Alabama
University Station
Birmingham 35294
205-934-7110

Sleep Disorders Center
The Children's Hospital
1600 7th Avenue South
Birmingham 35233
205-939-9386

Sleep Disorders Center (P)
Southeast Alabama Medical Center
P.O. Drawer 6987
Dothan 36302
205-793-8134

North Alabama Sleep Disorders Center (P)
Huntsville Hospital
101 Sivley Rd.
Huntsville 35801
205-533-8020

Sleep Disorders Lab (P)
Carraway Methodist Medical Center
1600 26th Street North
Birmingham 35234
205-226-6164

Knowllwood Sleep Disorders
Center (P)
Knowllwood Long Term Care
Hospital
P.O. Box 9813
Mobile 36691
205-666-7700

Sleep Disorders Center (P)
Mobile Infirmary Medical Center
P.O. Box 9813
Mobile 36691
205-431-2400

ARIZONA

Sleep Disorders Center
Good Samaritan Medical Center
1111 East McDowell Road
Phoenix 85006
602-239-5815

Sleep Disorders Center
University of Arizona
1501 North Campbell Avenue
Tucson 85724
602-626-6112

ARKANSAS

Sleep Disorders Diagnostic & Research Center
University of Arkansas for Medical Sciences
4301 West Markham, Slot 555
Little Rock 72205
501-661-5528

Sleep Disorders Center (P)
Baptist Medical Center
9601 I-630, Exit 7
Little Rock 72205
501-227-4750

Sleep Disorders Center (P)
St. Vincent Infirmary
No. 2 St. Vincent Circle
Little Rock 72205
501-660-3011

CALIFORNIA

San Diego Regional Sleep Disorders Center
Harbor View Medical Center
120 Elm Street
San Diego 92101
619-232-0537

Sleep Disorders Center
Scripps Clinic and Research Foundation
10666 N. Torrey Pines Rd.
La Jolla 92037
619-455-8087

UCLA Sleep Disorders Clinic
710 Westwood Plaza, Rm. 1184 RNRC
Los Angeles 90024
213-206-8005

Sleep Disorders Center
Holy Cross Hospital
15031 Rinaldi St.
Mission Hills 91345
818-898-4639

Sleep Disorders Center
U.C. Irvine Medical Center
101 City Drive South
Orange 92668
714-634-5777

Sleep Disorders Center
Sequoia Hospital
Whipple and Alameda
Redwood City 94062
415-367-5620

Sleep Disorders Program
Hoover Pavilion-2d floor
Stanford University Medical Center

Stanford 94305
415-723-6601

WMCA Sleep Disorders Center
Western Medical Center-Anaheim
1025 South Anaheim Blvd.
Anaheim 92805
714-491-1159

Sleep Disorders Clinic and Research Center
St. Mary's Hospital
450 Stanyan Street
San Francisco 94117
415-750-5579

Sleep Disorders Center
Torrance Memorial Hospital
3330 Lomita Blvd.
Torrance 90509
213-235-9110, ext. 2049

Sleep Apnea Center
Merritt-Peralta Medical Center
450 30th St.
Oakland 94609
415-451-4900, ext. 2273

Southern California Sleep Apnea Center
Lombard Medical Group
2230 Lynn Rd.
Thousand Oaks 91360
805-495-1066

Sleep Disorders Center (P)
Hoag Memorial Hospital Presbyterian
301 Newport Blvd.
Newport Beach 92663
714-760-5505

Sleep Disorders Center (P)
Downey Community Hospital
11500 Brookshire Avenue
Downey 90241
213-806-5280

Sleep Disorders Institute (P)
St. Jude Hospital and Rehabilitation Center
101 East Valencia Mesa Drive
Fullerton 92634
714-871-3280

Loma Linda Sleep Disorders Center (P)
V.A. Hospital (111P)
11201 Benton St.
Loma Linda 92354
714-825-7084, ext. 2703

Sleep Disorders Center (P)
The Hospital of the Good Samaritan
616 South Witmer Street
Los Angeles 90017
213-977-2206

Sleep Disorders Center (P)
Pomona Valley Community Hospital
1798 North Garey Avenue
Pomona 91767
714-623-8715, ext. 2135

Sleep Disorders Center (P)
San Jose Hospital
675 East Santa Clara Street
San Jose 95112
408-977-4445

Sleep Disorders Center (P)
South Coast Medical Center
31872 Coast Highway
South Laguna 92677
714-499-1311, ext. 2186

Sleep Disorders Center (P)
Pacific Presbyterian Medical Center
P.O. Box 7999
San Francisco 94120
415-923-3336

Sleep Disorders Center (P)
Grossmont District Hospital
P.O. Box 158
La Mesa 92044
619-465-0711

COLORADO

Sleep Disorders Center
Presbyterian Medical Center
1719 East 19th Avenue
Denver 80218
303-839-6447

Sleep Disorders Center
University of Colorado Health Sciences Center
700 Delaware St.
Denver 80204
303-592-7278

Porter Regional Sleep Disorders Center (P)
Porter Memorial Hospital
2525 South Downing St.
Denver 80210
303-744-6561

DISTRICT OF COLUMBIA

Sleep Disorders Center
Georgetown University Hospital
3800 Reservoir Road N.W.
Washington, D.C. 20007
202-625-2697, ext. 2020

FLORIDA

Sleep Disorders Center
Mt. Sinai Medical Center
4300 Alton Road
Miami Beach 33140
305-674-2613

Sleep-Related Breathing Disorders Center
Baptist Medical Center
800 Prudential Drive
Jacksonville 32207
904-393-2909

Sleep Disorders Center (P)
Good Samaritan Hospital
P.O. Box 3166
West Palm Beach 33402
305-655-5511

Sleep Disorders Center (P)
Tallahassee Medical Center, Inc.
Magnolia Drive and Miccosukee Rd.
Tallahassee 32308
904-681-1155

GEORGIA

Sleep Disorders Center
Northside Hospital
1000 Johnson Ferry Road
Atlanta 30342
404-851-8135

Sleep Disorders Center (P)
Memorial Medical Center, Inc.
P.O. Box 23089
Savannah 31403
912-356-8326

HAWAII

Sleep Disorders Center
Straub Clinic and Hospital
888 South King Street
Honolulu 96813
808-523-2311, ext. 8448

IDAHO

Idaho Sleep Disorders Center (P)
St. Luke's Regional Medical Center
190 East Bannock

Boise 83712
208-386-2440

ILLINOIS

Sleep Disorders Center
University of Chicago
5841 South Maryland, Box 425
Chicago 60637
312-962-1780

Sleep Disorders Center (P)
Rush-Presbyterian-St. Luke's
1753 West Congress Parkway
Chicago 60612
312-942-5440

Sleep Disorders Center
Methodist Medical Center of Illinois
221 N.E. Glen Oak
Peoria 61636
309-672-4966

Sleep Disorders Center (P)
Evanston Hospital
2650 Ridge Avenue
Evanston 60201
312-492-4983

Sleep Disorders Center (P)
Neurology Service
Veterans Hospital
Hines 60141
312-343-7200, ext. 2326

Sleep Disorders Clinic and Laboratory (P)
Carle Foundation Hospital
611 West Park St.
Urbana 61801
217-337-3364

INDIANA

Sleep Disorders Center
Winona Memorial Hospital
3232 North Meridian St.
Indianapolis 46208
317-927-2100

Sleep Disorders Laboratory (P)
St. Vincent Hospital
20001 West 86th St.
Indianapolis 46260
317-871-2152

Sleep/Wake Disorders Center (P)
Community Hospital of Indiana
1500 North Ritter Avenue
Indianapolis 46219
317-353-4275

Sleep Disorders Center (P)
St. Mary's Medical Center
3700 Washington Ave.
Evansville 47750
812-479-4257

Regional Sleep Studies Laboratory (P)
The Lutheran Hospital of Fort Wayne, Inc.
3024 Fairfield Avenue
Fort Wayne 46807
219-458-2001

Sleep Disorders Center (P)
Lafayette Home Hospital
2400 South St.
Lafayette 47903
317-447-6811

Sleep Disorders Diagnostic Center (P)
Methodist Hospital of Indiana
1801 N. Senate Blvd.
Indianapolis 46202
317-929-5710

IOWA

Mercy Hospital
Sleep Disorders Center

West Central Park at Marquette
Davenport 52804
319-383-1071

Sleep Disorders Center (P)
St. Luke's Hospital
1227 East Rushome St.
Davenport 52803
319-326-6740

Sleep Disorders Center (P)
Iowa Methodist Medical Center
1200 Pleasant St.
Des Moines 50308
515-283-6207

Sleep Disorders Center (P)
Department of Neurology
University of Iowa Hospitals and Clinics
Iowa City 52242
319-356-2571

KANSAS

Sleep Disorders Center (P)
Wesley Medical Center
550 North Hillside
Wichita 67214
319-688-2660

KENTUCKY

Sleep Disorders Center
Humana Hospital Audubon
One Audubon Plaza Drive
Louisville 40217
502-636-7459

Sleep Disorders Center (P)
St. Joseph's Hospital
One St. Joseph Drive
Lexington 40504
606-278-3436

LOUISIANA

Tulane Sleep Disorders Center
1415 Tulane Avenue
New Orleans 70112
504-587-7457

Sleep Disorders Center (P)
Willis-Knighton Medical Center
2600 Greenwood Rd.
Shreveport 71103
318-632-4823

MARYLAND

The Johns Hopkins University
Sleep Disorders Center
Francis Scott Key Medical Center
Baltimore 21224
301-955-0571

Maryland Sleep Diagnostic Center (P)
Ruxton Towers, Suite 211
8415 Bellona Ave.
Baltimore 21204
301-494-9773

MASSACHUSETTS

Sleep Disorders Center (P)
Boston University Medical Center
75 East Newton St.
Boston 02146
617-247-5206

Sleep Disorders Center (P)
Boston Children's Hospital
300 Longwood Ave.
Boston 02115
617-735-6242

Sleep Disorders Unit (P)
Beth Israel Hospital
330 Brookline Ave., KS430
Boston 02215
617-735-3237

Sleep/Wake Disorders Unit (P)
University of Massachusetts
55 Lake Avenue North
Worcester 01605
617-856-3802

MICHIGAN

Sleep Disorders Center
Henry Ford Hospital
2799 West Grand Blvd.
Detroit 48202
313-972-1800

Sleep Disorders Center
Ingham Medical Center
301 West Greenlawn Ave.
Lansing 48909
517-374-2510

Sleep/Wake Disorders Unit (P)
VA Medical Center
Southfield & Outer Drive
Allen Park 48101
313-562-6000

Sleep Disorders Clinic (P)
Catherine McAuley Health Center
P.O. Box 995
Ann Arbor 48106
313-572-3093

Sleep Disorders Center (P)
Taubman Center 1920/0316
1500 E. Medical Center Drive
Ann Arbor 48109
313-936-9068

Bloomfield Institute for Sleep (P)
Beaumont Hospital Medical Building
44199 Dequindre, Suite 403
Troy 48098
313-879-0707

Sleep Disorders Center (P)
Butterworth Hospital
100 Michigan St. NE
Grand Rapids 49503
616-774-1695

Sleep Disorders Center (P)
Traverse City Osteopathic Hospital
550 Munson Avenue
Traverse City 49684
616-922-8600

MINNESOTA

Sleep Disorders Center
Methodist Hospital
6500 Excelsior Blvd.
St. Louis Park 55426
612-932-6083

Sleep Disorders Center
Hennepin County Medical Center
Minneapolis 55415
612-347-6288

Sleep Disorders Center
Mayo Clinic
200 First St. SW
Rochester 55905
507-286-8900

Sleep Disorders Center (P)
Fairview Southdale Hospital
6401 France Avenue South
Edina 55435
612-924-5058

Sleep Disorders Center (P)
Abbott Northwestern Hospital
800 E. 28th St. at Chicago Ave.
Minneapolis 55407
612-874-4257

Sleep Diagnostic Center (P)
St. Joseph Hospital
69 West Exchange St.
St. Paul 55102
612-291-3682

Duluth Regional Sleep Disorders Center (P)
St. Mary's Medical Center
407 East Third St.
Duluth 55805
218-726-4543

MISSISSIPPI

Sleep Disorders Center
Division of Somnology
University of Mississippi
Jackson 39216
601-987-5552

Sleep Disorders Center (P)
Memorial Hospital at Gulfport
P.O. Box 1810
Gulfport 39501
601-865-3489

Sleep Disorders Center (P)
Forrest General Hospital
P.O. Box 16389
Hattiesburg 39401
601-264-4219

Gulf Coast Center for Sleep Disorders (P)
Gulf Coast Community Hospital
4642 West Beach Blvd.
Biloxi 39531
601-388-6711

MISSOURI

Sleep Disorders Center
St. Louis University Medical Center
1221 South Grand Blvd.
St. Louis 63104
314-577-8705

Sleep Disorders Center
Deaconess Hospital
6150 Oakland Ave.
St. Louis 63139
314-768-3100

Sleep Disorders Center
Research Medical Center
2316 East Meyer Blvd.
Kansas City 64132
816-276-4222

Sleep Disorders Center (P)
St. Mary's Hospital
28th St. and Main
Kansas City 64108
816-756-2651

Sleep Disorders Center (P)
L.E. Cox Medical Center
3801 S. National Avenue
Springfield 65807
417-885-6189

NEBRASKA

Sleep Physiology Center (P)
Lincoln General Hospital
2300 South 16th St.
Lincoln 68502
402-473-5338

Sleep Disorders Center (P)
Lutheran Medical Center
515 South 26th St.
Omaha 68103
402-536-6352

NEW HAMPSHIRE

Dartmouth-Hitchcock Sleep Disorders Center
Department of Psychiatry
Dartmouth Medical School
Hanover 03756
603-646-7534

Sleep-Wake Disorders Center (P)
Hampstead Hospital
East Road

Hampstead 03841
603-329-5311, ext. 240

NEW JERSEY

Sleep Disorders Center
Newark Beth Israel Medical Center
201 Lyons Avenue
Newark 07112
201-926-7597

NEW YORK

Sleep-Wake Disorders Center
Montefiore Hospital
111 East 210 St.
Bronx NY 10467
212-920-4841

Sleep Disorders Center
Columbia Presbyterian Medical Center
161 Forth Washington Ave.
New York, NY 10032
212-305-1860

Sleep Disorders Center
St. Mary's Hospital
89 Genesee St.
Rochester 14611
716-464-3391

Sleep Disorders Center
Department of Psychiatry
SUNY at Stony Brook
Stony Brook 11794
516-444-2916

Sleep-Wake Disorders Center
New York Hospital-Cornell Medical Center
21 Bloomingdale Rd.
White Plains 10605
914-997-5751

Sleep Disorders Center of Western New York (P)
Millard Fillmore Hospital
3 Gates Circle
Buffalo 14209
716-884-9253

Sleep Disorders Center (P)
Winthrop-University Hospital
259 First St.
Mineola 11501
516-663-2005

NORTH CAROLINA

Sleep Disorders Center (P)
Charlotte Memorial Hospital
P.O. Box 32861
Charlotte 28232
703-338-2121

Sleep Disorders Center (P)
Duke University Medical Center
P.O. Box 2905
Durham 27710
919-681-3344

Sleep Disorders Center (P)
The Moses H. Cone Memorial Hospital
1200 North Elm St.
Greensboro 27401
919-379-4406

NORTH DAKOTA

Sleep Disorders Center
St. Luke's Hospital
5th St. at Mills Avenue
Fargo 58122
701-280-5673

OHIO

Sleep/Wake Disorders Center
Miami Valley Hospital, Suite G200
Thirty Apple St.
Dayton 45409
513-220-2515

Sleep Disorders Center
Mercy Hospital of Fairfield
1275 East Kemper Rd.
Cincinnati 45246
513-671-3101

Sleep Disorders Center
Department of Neurology
Cleveland Clinic
Cleveland 44106
216-444-8732

Sleep Disorders Evaluation Center
Ohio State University Medical Center
473 West 12th Ave.
Columbus 43210
614-421-8296

Sleep Disorders Center
Bethesda Oak Hospital
619 Oak St.
Cincinnati 45206
513-569-6320

Northwest Ohio Sleep Disorders Center (P)
The Toledo Hospital
2142 North Cove Blvd.
Toledo 43606
419-471-5629

Sleep Disorders Center (P)
Southview Hospital
1997 Miamisburg-Centerville Rd.
Dayton 45459
513-439-6265

OKLAHOMA

Sleep Disorders Center
Presbyterian Hospital
N.E. 13th at Lincoln Blvd.
Oklahoma City 73104
405-271-6312

OREGON

Sleep Disorders Program
Good Samaritan Hospital
2222 N.W. Lovejoy St.
Portland 97210
503-229-8311

PENNSYLVANIA

Sleep Disorders Center
The Medical College of Pennsylvania
3300 Henry Avenue
Philadelphia 19129
215-842-4250

Sleep Disorders Center
Western Psychiatric Institute
38311 O'Hara St.
Pittsburgh 15213
412-624-2246

Sleep Disorders Center
Department of Neurology
Crozer-Chester Medical Center
Upland-Chester 19013
215-447-2689

Sleep Disorders Center
Jefferson Medical College
1015 Walnut St., Third Floor
Philadelphia 19107
215-928-6175

Sleep Disorders Center
Mercy Hospital of Johnstown
1127 Franklin St.
Johnstown 15905
814-533-1000

Sleep Disorders Center (P)
Hospital of the University of Pennsylvania
3400 Spruce St., 11 Gates
Philadelphia 19104
215-662-2833

SOUTH CAROLINA

Sleep Disorders Center (P)
Baptist Medical Center
Taylor at Marion Street
Columbia 29220
803-771-5557

Sleep Disorders Center (P)
Spartanburg Regional Medical Center
101 East Wood St.
Spartanburg 29303
803-591-6524

SOUTH DAKOTA

Sleep Disorders Center (P)
Sioux Valley Hospital
1100 South Euclid
Sioux Falls 57117
605-333-6302

Rushmore Diagnostic Center for Sleep Disorders (P)
Rushmore National Health Systems
353 Fairmont Blvd.
P.O. Box 6000
Rapid City 57709
605-341-8010

TENNESSEE

BMH Sleep Disorders Center
Baptist Memorial Hospital
899 Madison Ave.
Memphis 38146
901-522-5704

Sleep Disorders Center
Saint Thomas Hospital
P.O. Box 380
Nashville 37202
615-386-2068

Sleep Disorders Center
St. Mary's Medical Center
Oak Hill Ave.
Knoxville 37917
615-971-6011

Sleep Disorders Center (P)
Ft. Sanders Regional Medical Center
19001 West Clinch Ave.
Knoxville 37916
615-971-1375

TEXAS

Sleep-Wake Disorders Center
Presbyterian Hospital
8200 Walnut Hill Lane
Dallas 75231
214-696-8563

Sleep Disorders Center
All Saints Episcopal Hospital
1400 8th Ave.
Fort Worth 76104
817-927-6120

Sleep Disorders Center
Department of Psychiatry
Baylor College of Medicine
Houston 77030
713-799-4886

Humana Sleep Disorders Center
1303 McCullough
Suite 447
San Antonio 78212
512-223-4057

Sleep Disorders Center
Scott and White Clinic
2401 South 31st St.
Temple 76508
817-774-2554

Sleep Disorders Center
Sun Towers Hospital
1801 North Oregon

El Paso 79902
915-532-6281

Sleep Disorders Center (P)
Sam Houston Memorial Hospital
8300 Waterbury, Suite 350
Houston 77055
713-973-6483

Sleep Disorders Center (P)
Pasadena Bayshore Medical Center
4000 Spencer Highway
Pasadena 71504
713-944-6666

The Center for Sleep Disorders (P)
Lubbock General Hospital
P.O. Box 5980
Lubbock 79417
806-743-2020

West Texas Regional Sleep Disorders Center (P)
Odessa Women's and Children's Hospital
P.O. Box 4859
Odessa 79760
915-334-8352

Center for Sleep Disorders (P)
Department of Psychiatry UTHSC
7703 Floyd Curl Drive
San Antonio 78284
512-691-7531

UTAH

Intermountain Sleep Disorders Center
LDS Hospital
325 89th Avenue
Salt Lake City 84143
801-321-3417

Sleep Disorders Center (P)
Utah Neurological Clinic
1055 North 300 West, Suite 400
Provo 84604
801-379-7400

VIRGINIA

Sleep Disorders Center
Norfolk General Hospital
600 Gresham Drive
Norfolk 23507
804-628-3322

Sleep Disorders Center (P)
Community Hospital of Roanoke Valley
P.O. Box 12946
Roanoke 24029
703-985-8435

Sleep Disorders Center (P)
Chippenham Hospital
7101 Jahnke Road
Richmond 23232
804-320-3911, ext. 173

WASHINGTON

Sleep Disorders Center
Providence Medical Center
500 17th Avenue, C-34008
Seattle 98124
206-326-5366

WEST VIRGINIA

Sleep Disorders Center (P)
Charleston Area Medical Center
P.O. Box 1393
Charleston 23525
304-348-7507

WISCONSIN

Sleep Disorders Center
Gundersen Clinic, Ltd.
1836 South Avenue
La Crosse 54601
608-782-7300

Milwaukee Regional Sleep
Disorders Center (P)
Columbia Hospital
20205 East Newport Avenue
Milwaukee 53211
414-961-4650

Sleep Disorders Center Box 1997 (P)
Children's Hospital of Wisconsin
1700 West Wisconsin Avenue
Milwaukee 53201
414-931-4016

Sleep Disorders Center (P)
University Hospital & Clinics
600 Highland Avenue
Madison 53792
608-263-7050

Sleep/Wake Disorders Center
(P)
St. Mary's Hospital
2323 North Lake Drive
Milwaukee 53201
414-225-8032

REFERENCES

CHAPTER 1 *(Caffeine)*

"Caffeine and You," *Prevention,* June 1985.
A concise summary of caffeine's health effects.

Gilbert, Richard. *Caffeine, The Most Popular Stimulant.* Edgmont, Pa.: Chelsea House, 1986.

Goulart, Frances. *The Caffeine Book: A User's and Abuser's Guide,* New York: Dodd, Mead, 1984.
Two popular-level book-length discussions.

Dews, P.B. (ed.). *Caffeine Perspective from Recent Research,* New York: Springer-Verlag, 1984.
First-rate for those with a serious scientific interest in caffeine.

CHAPTER 2 *(Sugar)*

Bennion, Lynn. *Hypoglycemia: Fact or Fad?* New York: Crown, 1983
A well-written statement of the establishment viewpoint.

Fredericks, Carlton, *New Low Blood Sugar and You.* New York: Perigee, 1985.
An update on his earlier classic *Low Blood Sugar and You,* by the most influential advocate of diet-induced hypoglycemia.

Chalew, Stuart, Judith McLauglin, James Mersey, et. al. "The Use of Plasma Epinephrine Response in the Diagnosis of Idiopathic Postprandial Syndrome," *Journal of the American Medical Association,* 251 (Feb. 3, 1984), 612-615.
The best scientific study that supports the view that hypoglycemia is real and that adrenalin discharge rather than low blood sugar per se is the main cause of symptoms.

CHAPTER 3 *(Vitamins and Minerals)*

The following references cover the contending schools of thought about the role of nutrition.

Conservative

Herbert, V. and S. Barrett. *Vitamins and "Health" Foods: The Great American Hustle.* Philadelphia: George F. Stickley Co., 1984.

Drs. Herbert and Barrett are the leading crusaders against unscientific and improper nutritional claims.

Nutrition Forum (George F. Stickley Co., 210 W. Washington Square, Philadelphia, Pa. 19106).

A monthly newsletter about nutrition edited by Dr. Stephen Barrett.

Progressive

Nutrition Action (Center for Science in the Public Interest, 1501 16th St, N.W., Washington, D.C. 20036).

An interesting and reliable newsletter. Recommended.

Brody, J. *Jane Brody's Nutrition Book,* New York: Bantam, 1981.

The best of its kind, by *The New York Times'* health reporter.

American Health

A general health-oriented magazine, well-written and reliable.

Orthomolecular

Prevention (Rodale Press, Emmaus, Pa).

The leading popularly written nutrition-oriented magazine, *Prevention* is more in the mainstream than in years past, but it remains respectful of orthomolecular opinions.

Fredericks, Carlton. *Carlton Fredericks' Nutrition Guide for the Prevention and Cause of Common Ailments and Diseases.* New York: Simon & Schuster, 1982.

A good summary of the views of one of the most persuasive advocates of the power of nutrition.

SOURCES FOR PROFESSIONAL CONSULTATION

Your county medical society can provide a list of physicians who are interested in nutrition and who maintain the respect of their colleagues.

American Society for Clinical Nutrition, 9650 Rockville Pike, Bethesda, Md. 20814.

The leading organization of professional nutritionists. Predominantly conservative, but includes many progressives.

American College of Nutrition, P.O. Box 831, White Plains, N.Y. 10602.

Definitely mainstream and academic, but its journal and membership reflect a progressive sympathy on issues such as the effect of vitamin and mineral deficiencies on health.

American Dietetic Association, 430 N. Michigan Ave., Chicago, Ill. 60611.

The organization of registered dietitians. All schools are represented, but the official line tends to follow that set by organized medicine.

Academy of Orthomolecular Medicine, 2229 Broad St., Regina, Sask., S4P 1Y7.

Formerly the Academy of Orthomolecular Psychiatry, this is the leading professional organization advocating megavitamin treatments.

CHAPTER 4 *(Food Allergy)*

Randolph, Theron and R. Moss. *An Alternative Approach to Allergies.* New York: Lippincott, 1979.

Dr. Randolph is one of the originators of the controversial specialty of clinical ecology.

Mandell, M. *Dr. Mandell's 5-Day Allergy Relief System.* New York: Pocket Books, 1979.

Easier reading than Randolph's version but the same perspective. Note, however, that Dr. Mandell recommends a four-day fast taking only water. I do not think this is safe for routine use.

Malesky, G., "Find Your Food Foes and Discover Relief," *Prevention,* April 1986.

A nice summary of recent scientific research.

May, C. "Food Allergies: Lessons from the Past," *Journal of Allergy and Clinical Immunology 69* (March 1982): 255-59.

A scholarly summary of the view that food allergies are probably "all in your head."

"Position Statement on Clinical Ecology," American College of Allergists, 800 East Northwest Highway, Suite 101, Mount Prospect, Ill. 60056.

A skeptical view of food allergy and clinical ecology by a leading allergy society.

Brostoff, Jonathan and Stephen Challacombe. *Food Allergy and Intolerance.* London: Bailliere Tindall, 1987.

A 1000+ page book written for physicians and scientists but accessible to the motivated lay person. The most comprehensive medical textbook on food allergy, unique in that it provides respectful audience to both traditional and clinical ecology viewpoints.

PROFESSIONAL REFERRALS

American Academy of Allergy and Clinical Immunology, 611 Wells Avenue, Milwaukee, Wis. 53202.

American College of Allergy, 800 East Northwest Highway, Suite 101, Mount Prospect, Ill. 60056.

These are the two leading allergy professional societies.

American Academy of Environmental Medicine, P.O. Box 16106, Denver, Colo. 80216.

This is the main professional organization for physicians who believe undetected food allergy is common and important.

CHAPTER 5 *(Candida Yeast Theory)*

Truss, C.O. *The Missing Diagnosis.* Birmingham, Ala.: C. Orian Truss, 1982.

Dr. Truss is the originator of the candida yeast theory.

Crook, W. *The Yeast Connection.* Jackson, Tenn.: Professional Books, 1985.

Dr. Crook is a leading exponent of the candida theory.

"Position Paper on the Candida Yeast Theory," American Academy of Allergy and Immunology, 611 E. Wells St., Milwaukee, Wisc. 53202.

A skeptical evaluation of the scientific evidence pertaining to the candida theory.

CHAPTER 6 *(Stress)*

Selye, Hans. *The Stress of Life,* rev. New York: McGraw-Hill, 1976.
A nontechnical discussion of the scientific basis for understanding stress by the father of stress sciences.

Benson, Herbert. *Beyond the Relaxation Response.* New York: Berkley Books, 1985.
A leading stress researcher, Benson provides a philosophical and practical overview with emphasis on simple techniques for eliciting the relaxation response.

Friedman, M. and R. Rosenmann. *Type A Behavior and Your Heart.* New York: Fawcett Crest, 1974.
The original book about the Type A "hurry sickness."

Aronson, S. and Michael Mascia. *The Stress Management Workbook.* New York: Appleton-Century-Crofts, 1979.

Charlesworth, Edward and Ronald Nathan. *Stress Management: A Comprehensive Guide to Wellness.* New York: Atheneum, 1985.

Girdano, D., G. Everly. *Controlling Stress and Tension: A Holistic Approach.* NJ: Prentice-Hall, Englewood Cliffs, 1979.

Pelletier, Kenneth, *Mind as Healer, Mind as Slayer: A Holistic Approach to Preventing Stress Disorders.* Delacorte, NY 1977.

Tavris, Carol. "Coping With Anxiety," *Science Digest,* February 1986.
A nice magazine-article-length summary of the state of the art.

Psychology Today
The best of the popular psychology-oriented magazines.

RELAXATION TAPES

There are dozens of good tapes that will teach you various relaxation techniques. Consider selections from the catalogs of Yes! Bookshop, 1035 31st St., NW, Washington, DC 20007; *Medical Self-Care* magazine, P.O. Box 1000, Point Reyes, CA 94956; or *New Age,* Box 220, Alliston, MA 02134.

CHAPTER 7

Erikson, Erik. *The Life Cycle Completed: A Review.* New York: Norton, 1982.
Erikson's work provides one basis for current thinking about the predictable crises of psychological development in childhood through to old age. This volume is a very brief but somewhat technical summary. More popularly written are his earlier books, including *Childhood and Society* (1950), *Identity: Youth and Crisis* (1968).

Sheehy, Gail. *Pathfinders.* New York: William Morrow, 1981.
Sheehy, Gail. *Passages.* New York: Dutton, 1974.
Sheehy's best-selling works apply Erickson's concepts to current American life in a popular style.

CHAPTER 8 *(Depression)*

Burns, David. *Feeling Good.* New York: New American Library, 1980.
A leader of the cognitive school of psychotherapy, Dr. Burns emphasizes identifying and changing negative feelings and attitudes as the key to sound mental health. Contains an excellent self-assessment scale for depression, The Beck Depression Inventory.

Gold, Mark. *The Good News About Depression.* New York: Villard, 1987.
Dr. Gold is a leading exponent of the view that depression is a biochemical disease.

Papolos, Dimitri and Janice Papolos. *Overcoming Depression.* New York: Harper & Row, 1987.
Up-to-date, comprehensive, readable, and reliable.

CHAPTER 9 *(Sleep)*

Lamberg, Lynne. *The American Medical Association Guide to Better Sleep.* New York: Random House, 1984.
A comprehensive introduction to sleep problems. The writing is exceptionally clear.

Maxmen, Jerrold. *A Good Night's Sleep.* New York: Norton, 1981.
Regestein, Quentin and James Rechs. *Sound Sleep,* New York: Simon & Schuster, 1980.

Well-written guides to better sleep.

Guilleminault, C. *Sleeping and Waking Disorders: Indications and Techniques.* Menlo Park, Calif.: Addison-Wesley, 1982.
A classic textbook for physicians.

CHAPTER 10 *(Situational Fatigue)*

Burns, David. *Feeling Good.* New York: New American Library, 1980.
The cognitive approach is particularly apt for situations in which tiredness is your body's way of saying no.

Padus, Emrika. *The Complete Guide to Your Emotions and Your Health.* Emmaus, Pa.: Rodale Press, 1986.
Not as critical as some might wish, but very broad-ranging and very good on the kind of commonsense advice that helps in situational fatigue.

CHAPTER 11 *(Mind/Body Interface)*

American Psychiatric Association. *The Diagnostic and Statistical Manual,* vol. 3. Washington, D.C., 1980.
A readable, relatively nontechnical discussion of the major psychiatric diagnoses.

Locke, Steven and Douglas Colligan. *The Healer Within: The New Medicine of Mind and Body.* New York: Dutton, 1986.
An excellent presentation of the view that mind and body ills are intimately related.

CHAPTER 12 *(Medicines and Drugs of Abuse)*

Key references appear in the text of the chapter.

Goodwin, Donald. *Alcoholism, The Facts.* New York: Oxford University Press, 1981.

Ausubel, David. *What Every Well-Informed Person Should Know About Drug Addiction.* Chicago: Nelson-Hall, 1980.

Cohen, Sidney. *The Substance Abuse Problem.* New York: Haworth Press, 1981.

CHAPTER 13 *(Environment and Fatigue)*

Light

John Ott. *Health and Light.* New York: Pocket Books, 1983.

A popular discussion of the hazards and benefits of different forms of light. Not fully accepted by scientists, but definitely an important influence on current research.

I have not encountered a good, scientifically acceptable, popular book describing current research on light and health. If you suspect a problem that your local physicians cannot address, your doctor might contact a national center such as the National Institute of Mental Health, 9000 Rockville, Pike, Bethesda, Md. 20205 (Att: Dr. Norman Rosenthal); Sleep and Mood Disorder Laboratory, L 469, Oregon Health Sciences University, Portland, Or. 97201 (Att: Dr. Alfred Lewy); Department of Nutrition, Massachusetts Institute of Technology, Cambridge, Mass. 02139 (Att: Dr. Richard Wurtman); Department of Medicine, Brigham and Women's Hospital, 221 Longwood Avenue, Boston, Mass. 02115 (Att: Dr. C.A. Czeisler)

The main source of full spectrum very bright lights is the Duro-test company of North Bergen, N.J. However, as of this writing, their sale is restricted to researchers who study the effect of light on fatigue, depression, sleep problems, and other illnesses. (Duro-test sells a normal brightness light that simulates the full spectrum of the sun. However, this is not as bright as the lights being used to treat seasonal depression or sleep disorders.)

Climate

Soyka, Fred and Alan Edmonds. *The Ion Effect,* New York: Bantam, 1978.

A readable but overenthusiastic account of the relationship between ions in the air and how people feel.

The American Institute of Medical Climatology, 1023 Welsh Road, Philadelphia, Pa. 19115. Tel. 215-673-8368.

A professional organization for those seriously interested in climate and health.

Workplace and Indoor Air

Makower, Joel. *Office Hazards: How Your Job Can Make You Sick.* Washington, D.C.: Tilden Press, 1981.

One of the very best discussions of all aspects of the physical and psychological environment in white-collar office settings.

Stelman, Jeanne and Susan Daum. *Work is Dangerous to Your Health: A Handbook of Health Hazards in the Workplace and What You Can Do About Them.* New York: Vintage Books, 1971.
Somewhat dated but relatively clear and easy to use guide to blue-collar and industrial health and safety hazards.

Chemical Environment

Legator, Marvin, Barbara Harper, and Michael Scott. *The Health Detective's Handbook: A Guide to the Investigation of Environmental Hazards by Nonprofessionals.* Baltimore: Johns Hopkins University Press, 1985.
A practical overview of all kinds of pollution problems, with a decent bibliography.

Randolph, Theron and Ralph Moss. *An Alternative Approach to Allergies.* New York: Bantam, 1980.
A clinical ecology perspective by the founder of this specialty. A minority viewpoint, but the first to pay serious attention to patients such as Ed, the "allergic to everything" chemist described in this chapter.

"Position Statement on Clinical Ecology," American College of Allergists, 800 East Northwest Highway, Suite 101, Mount Prospect, Ill. 60056, 1986.
A skeptical view of the chemical-sensitivity theory of clinical ecology by a leading allergy society.

Carson, Rachel. *Silent Spring.* Houghton Mifflin, Boston: 1962.
Out-of-date perhaps, but still the classic presentation of responsible concern about the future of our chemical environment.

Science, April 17, 1987, pages 267-300.
A series of intelligent articles about assessing the risk of potential environmental hazards. Includes an examination of the problem of environmental chemicals which argues that there is little danger.

Golos, Natalie and Frances Golbitz. *Coping With Your Allergies.* New York: Simon & Schuster, 1979.
A practical guide about pollution in the home, heavily flavored with clinical ecology perspective.

CHEMICAL TESTING

If your doctor feels you might benefit from testing your blood or urine for pesticide or other chemical exposures, several reputable laboratories accept samples by mail. I use and have been satisfied with Envirohealth Systems, Inc., 990 North Bowser Rd., Richardson, Tex. 75081; Tel. 800-558-0069.

CHAPTERS 14 & 15 *(Physical Illness)*

General

Brody, Jane. *New York Times Guide to Personal Health.* New York: Times Books, 1976.

Foster, Daniel. *A Layman's Guide to Modern Medicine.* New York: Simon and Schuster, 1980.

Good Housekeeping Health And Medical Guide. New York: Hearst, 1980.

Arthritis and Autoimmune Problems

Fries, James. *Arthritis: A Comprehensive Guide.* Reading, Mass.: Addison-Wesley, 1979 .

Epstein-Barr Virus

Physicians seeking a list of specialists in the forefront of E-B virus research might write to the Division of Medical Virology, Building 10, Room 11N-113, National Institutes of Health, Bethesda, Md. 20205.

National CEBV Syndrome Association, PO Box 230108, Portland, Ore. 97223.

This is the national support group for people diagnosed as having the chronic Epstein-Barr virus syndrome.

Gastrointestinal

Nugent, Nancy. *How to Get Along with Your Stomach.* Boston: Little, Brown, 1978.

Heart Disease

The American Heart Association Heartbook. New York: Dutton, 1980.

Lung Disease

Petty, Thomas and Louise Nett. *For Those Who Live and Breathe: A Manual for Patients with Emphysema and Chronic Bronchitis.* Springfield, Ill.: Charles C. Thomas, 1984.

Young, Stuart, Susan Schulman, and Martin Schulman. *The Asthma Handbook.* New York: Bantam, 1985.

Menopause

Cutler, Winnifred, Celso-Ramon Garcia, and David Edwards. *Menopause.* New York: Norton, 1983.

Budoff, Penny. *Menopause.* New York: Putnam, 1983.

HERS Foundation, 422 Bryn Mawr Avenue, Bala Cynwyd, Pa. 19004
A self-help organization for women whose fatigue and other symptoms might be related to menopause.

Premenstrual Syndrome

Dalton, Katerina. *Once a Month.* Claremont, Calif.: Hunter House, 1983.
The most influential (and controversial) PMS expert, Dr. Dalton emphasizes the use of natural progesterone in treating PMS.

Laurensen, N. and E. Stukane. *PMS: Premenstrual Syndrome and You.* New York: Simon & Schuster, 1984.
An holistic approach; discusses a broad array of treatments.

Witt, Reni. *PMS.* New York: Stein & Day, 1983.
A wide-ranging survey of treatment choices, well balanced between enthusiasm and skepticism.

PMS Action, PO Box 9326, Madison, Wis. 53715; Tel: 608-274- 6688.
A self-help organization, PMS Action provides a newsletter and resources for women with PMS.

Thyroid

Barnes, B. and L. Galton. *Hypothyroidism: The Unsuspected Illness.* New York: Harper & Row, 1976.
Provides the unorthodox view that low thyroid is an epidemic but unappreciated disease.

Wood, L., D. Cooper and E. Ridgway. *Your Thyroid.* Boston: Houghton Mifflin, 1982.

A good summary of the mainstream view by leading specialists in thyroid disorders.

INDEX